DEADLY DISEASES AND EPIDEMICS

PLAGUE

DEADLY DISEASES AND EPIDEMICS

Anthrax

Campylobacteriosis

Cholera

Escherichia coli Infections

Gonorrhea

Hepatitis

Herpes

HIV/AIDS

Influenza

Lyme Disease

Mad Cow Disease (Bovine Spongiform Encephalopathy)

Malaria

Meningitis

Mononucleosis

Plague

Polio

SARS

Smallpox

Streptococcus (Group A)

Syphilis

Toxic Shock Syndrome

Tuberculosis

Typhoid Fever

West Nile Virus

DEADLY DISEASES AND EPIDEMICS

PLAGUE

Donald Emmeluth

CONSULTING EDITOR
The Late I. Edward Alcamo
The Late Distinguished Teaching Professor of Microbiology,
SUNY Farmingdale

FOREWORD BY
David Heymann
World Health Organization

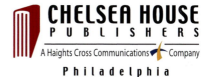

CHELSEA HOUSE
PUBLISHERS
A Haights Cross Communications Company
Philadelphia

Dedication

We dedicate the books in the DEADLY DISEASES AND EPIDEMICS series to Ed Alcamo, whose wit, charm, intelligence, and commitment to biology education were second to none.

CHELSEA HOUSE PUBLISHERS

VP, NEW PRODUCT DEVELOPMENT Sally Cheney
DIRECTOR OF PRODUCTION Kim Shinners
CREATIVE MANAGER Takeshi Takahashi
MANUFACTURING MANAGER Diann Grasse

Staff for Plague

EXECUTIVE EDITOR Tara Koellhoffer
ASSOCIATE EDITOR Beth Reger
ASSISTANT EDITOR Margaret Brierton
PRODUCTION EDITOR Noelle Nardone
PHOTO EDITOR Sarah Bloom
SERIES DESIGNER Terry Mallon
COVER DESIGNER Keith Trego
LAYOUT 21st Century Publishing and Communications, Inc.

A Haights Cross Communications ✦ Company

http://www.chelseahouse.com

First Printing

1 3 5 7 9 8 6 4 2

Library of Congress Cataloging-in-Publication Data

Emmeluth, Donald.
   Plague/Donald Emmeluth
      p. cm.—(Deadly diseases and epidemics)
Includes bibliographical references and index.
   ISBN 0-7910-7306-8 — ISBN 0-7910-8345-4 (pbk.)
   1. Plague. I. Title. II. Series.
RA644.P7E47 2004
616.9'232—dc22

                                                        2004010102

All links and web addresses were checked and verified to be correct at the time of publication. Because of the dynamic nature of the web, some addresses and links may have changed since publication and may no longer be valid.

Table of Contents

Foreword

In the 1960s, many of the infectious diseases that had terrorized generations were tamed. After a century of advances, the leading killers of Americans both young and old were being prevented with new vaccines or cured with new medicines. The risk of death from pneumonia, tuberculosis (TB), meningitis, influenza, whooping cough, and diphtheria declined dramatically. New vaccines lifted the fear that summer would bring polio, and a global campaign was on the verge of eradicating smallpox worldwide. New pesticides like DDT cleared mosquitoes from homes and fields, thus reducing the incidence of malaria, which was present in the southern United States and which remains a leading killer of children worldwide. New technologies produced safe drinking water and removed the risk of cholera and other water-borne diseases. Science seemed unstoppable. Disease seemed destined to all but disappear.

But the euphoria of the 1960s has evaporated.

The microbes fought back. Those causing diseases like TB and malaria evolved resistance to cheap and effective drugs. The mosquito developed the ability to defuse pesticides. New diseases emerged, including AIDS, Legionnaires, and Lyme disease. And diseases which had not been seen in decades re-emerged, as the hantavirus did in the Navajo Nation in 1993. Technology itself actually created new health risks. The global transportation network, for example, meant that diseases like West Nile virus could spread beyond isolated regions and quickly become global threats. Even modern public health protections sometimes failed, as they did in 1993 in Milwaukee, Wisconsin, resulting in 400,000 cases of the digestive system illness cryptosporidiosis. And, more recently, the threat from smallpox, a disease believed to be completely eradicated, has returned along with other potential bioterrorism weapons such as anthrax.

The lesson is that the fight against infectious diseases will never end.

In our constant struggle against disease, we as individuals have a weapon that does not require vaccines or drugs, and that is the warehouse of knowledge. We learn from the history of science that "modern" beliefs can be wrong. In this series of books, for example, you will learn that diseases like syphilis were once thought to be caused by eating potatoes. The invention of the microscope set science on the right path. There are more positive lessons from history. For example, smallpox was eliminated by vaccinating everyone who had come in contact with an infected person. This "ring" approach to smallpox control is still the preferred method for confronting an outbreak, should the disease be intentionally reintroduced.

At the same time, we are constantly adding new drugs, new vaccines, and new information to the warehouse. Recently, the entire human genome was decoded. So too was the genome of the parasite that causes malaria. Perhaps by looking at the microbe and the victim through the lens of genetics we will be able to discover new ways to fight malaria, which remains the leading killer of children in many countries.

Because of advances in our understanding of such diseases as AIDS, entire new classes of anti-retroviral drugs have been developed. But resistance to all these drugs has already been detected, so we know that AIDS drug development must continue.

Education, experimentation, and the discoveries that grow out of them are the best tools to protect health. Opening this book may put you on the path of discovery. I hope so, because new vaccines, new antibiotics, new technologies, and, most importantly, new scientists are needed now more than ever if we are to remain on the winning side of this struggle against microbes.

David Heymann
Executive Director
Communicable Diseases Section
World Health Organization
Geneva, Switzerland

1

Historical Overview

The word *plague* is defined as a dangerous disease that spreads rapidly and often causes death. It is synonymous with a cause of suffering or harm. If we call it the bubonic plague or, better yet, the Black Death, the disease becomes a series of well-known historical events that resulted in the death and suffering of millions of people. But this is not just an event of the past. Each year, in the United States, between 20 and 40 individuals are infected with the organism that causes bubonic plague, *Yersinia pestis*. New Mexico alone averages 7 to 8 cases a year. Bubonic plague occurs in more than 20 countries worldwide, with an average of more than 2,000 total cases.

The following is a fictionalized version of an event that occurred in New York City in November 2002. The names of the hospital, doctors, and hospital administrators are accurate. It should be remembered that both the city and country were still extremely concerned about bioterrorism in the wake of September 11, 2001, and the anthrax attacks in the fall of the same year. The death of several people from anthrax had everyone on edge, and none more so than the medical community.

THE TRIP

They had saved for months in order to make the trip. They had been looking forward to seeing New York City in the fall. Although Santa Fe, New Mexico, was a medium-sized city, it lacked the character and excitement of New York City. And there was also Ground Zero. The World Trade Center destruction area was a magnet for many, and husband and wife John Tull and Lucinda Marker were among those who felt drawn to make the pilgrimage.

Both John and Lucinda came down with fevers and flu-like symptoms at the same time, shortly before their trip. They took some over-the-counter medication and drank plenty of fluids. They were determined that this little discomfort was not going to stop their trip. And so, congested and feverish, they boarded the plane and winged their way to the Big Apple.

New York City in the fall can be an imposing place. Winds blowing between the buildings and down the streets create a windchill factor that shocks visitors from the Southwest. Yet, John and Lucinda did not feel terribly cold because their fevers had not abated. Unfortunately, John was feeling weak and had difficulty walking for any length of time. Lucinda felt a swelling in her groin region, and the areas behind her knees and in her armpits were feeling tender and also seemed swollen. Both agreed that they needed to contact a doctor. Before they left Santa Fe, they had had their family doctor provide them with the name of a physician they could contact in the area of the city where they would be staying. When they contacted Dr. Ronald Primas and described their symptoms, he made an immediate appointment to have them examined. He was concerned that they might have smallpox, West Nile virus, anthrax, possibly the plague or—he hoped—just the flu. Once Dr. Primas saw the couple and examined Lucinda, however, it was clear that she probably had bubonic plague. John's symptoms were also consistent with that diagnosis. That initial diagnosis was strengthened when the couple mentioned that a rat on their property had tested positive for the plague back in July. The bacteria that cause the plague are constantly present in low concentrations in fleas that live on rats, squirrels, and domesticated dogs and cats throughout the Southwest.

Dr. Primas referred the couple to Beth Israel Medical Center. The patients were placed in isolation, and the New York City Department of Health was notified. None of the doctors in the hospital had ever seen a case of plague.

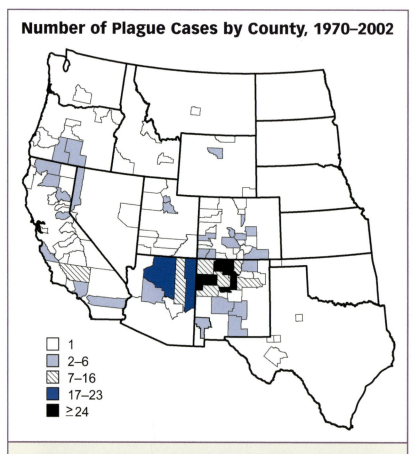

Number of Plague Cases by County, 1970–2002

Legend:
- 1
- 2–6
- 7–16
- 17–23
- ≥24

Figure 1.1 Although many people think of plague as something out of the Middle Ages, it is actually endemic (always present to some extent), especially in the Southwest of the United States (although it is rarely deadly as it was in medieval times).

Though the form of plague that the couple had was not contagious, it could become so if not treated within the next few days. Health Department personnel gave the couple a new diagnostic test that involved checking their blood for the presence of certain types of protective proteins called **antibodies**. (More information about this test will be presented in Chapter 9.) This test was part of a series of new tests developed since the September 11 attacks. The tests came back positive for bubonic plague. It was clear that the couple had contracted the disease back home in New Mexico. It was also clear that this was not an instance of bioterrorism. After a few days of antibiotic treatment, Lucinda was released from the hospital and John was making a slow, modest recovery.

THE PRESENT-DAY PLAGUE

It may seem hard to believe that a disease that presumably caused the death of millions during the 14th, 15th, and 16th centuries is still active in the United States in the 21st century. In actuality, between 10 and 30 people in the United States are infected yearly. Plague appears in about 15 states, with most cases occurring in the West (Figure 1.1). According to the Centers for Disease Control and Prevention (CDC), between 1,000 and 3,000 people are infected annually worldwide. Dr. Thomas Frieden, health commissioner of New York City, indicates that half of all cases in the United States originate in New Mexico in Santa Fe County, the county where Lucinda and John live. Fleas that attach themselves to wild animals carry the disease organism. They are the **vectors**, or carriers of the disease. The large rodent population in Santa Fe County is the suggested cause of the large number of infections in the area.

THE BLACK DEATH

Historical records suggest that a plague began in Egypt in A.D. 541, affecting a significant portion of the known world. It is estimated that 50 to 60% of the population died from that **pandemic** (a worldwide epidemic). The second great plague pandemic began in 1346. It became known as the Black Death, or the Great Pestilence, because of the distinctive symptoms that the disease produced. Symptoms included a swelling of regional lymph nodes in the groin, behind the knees, and under the arms. Ulcerations were common on the skin, but the most distinctive feature was the dark color beneath the skin where blood vessels had ruptured, turning the skin black in those areas. Hence, the disease was given the name the "Black Death."

Within five years, more than 13 million people had died in China, and, in Europe, the disease may have killed three out of every four people it infected. The plague continued over the next 300 years, killing between 20 and 30 million people in Europe. (It seemed to disappear around 1670.)

Historical records indicate that a third pandemic began in China in the mid-1850s. Its distribution seems to have paralleled the expansion of the Chinese Empire. As Chinese troops moved into regions of Burma, India, and Hong Kong, the plague organism moved with them. It continued to spread aboard steamships that went to European and American ports. The plague ended around 1910.

Whenever and however the plague organism became established in the United States, it spread into the western and southwestern portions of the country. Most human cases occur in northern New Mexico, northern Arizona, southern Colorado, California, southern Oregon, and far western Nevada. Worldwide since 1989, human plague cases have been reported in 11 countries. More than 370 cases were reported from Vietnam and 180 from Madagascar. Brazil has had more than 26 cases and Bolivia more than 7. Bubonic plague continues to be **endemic** (constantly present, though with few cases) in many areas of the world.

THE CAUSE

The causative agent of bubonic plague was identified by Alexander Yersin in 1894. He recognized that it was caused by a bacterium that ultimately was named after him, *Yersinia pestis*. We will explore the nature of this bacterium in greater detail in Chapter 2.

Yersin, who worked for the Pasteur Institute in France, developed a treatment that was marginally effective in combating the disease and was the first to suggest that rats and fleas were responsible for transmission of the organism during the **epidemic** of 1894 in Hong Kong.

In an attempt to produce a vaccine to protect people against bubonic plague, Yersin inoculated horses with increasing doses of the plague organism that had been killed by heat. Yersin's team of assistants then had to remove blood from the horses. They separated the fluid portion (the **plasma**) from the blood cells and inactivated the various proteins that cause blood to clot. The plasma with the clotting factors removed is known as the **serum** and is the portion of the blood that contains the antibodies against the plague organisms. These antibodies are designed to neutralize the protein toxins released by the bacteria. The vaccine varied in quality, and horses frequently died from the process. Yersin had hoped to produce more than 7,000 doses of the vaccine but was persuaded to go to India with only his available vaccine doses.

In 1897, Alexander Yersin left the Pasteur Institute and entered Bombay Harbor with 700 doses of his antiplague serum. After two months of treating patients, nearly half had died. A new batch of serum from France increased the survival rate to 80%. However, the Bombay government began to restrict Yersin's access to patients. He was allowed to inject only those patients who were already too far advanced in their illness to be helped. When the Pasteur Institute recalled him, Yersin left Bombay without regret.

The symptoms of bubonic plague usually begin to emerge within one to seven days after a person is bitten by an infected flea. Symptoms usually include fever and swelling in the regional lymph nodes in the groin, armpit, or neck regions. There are many additional symptoms that may occur (Figure 1.2). The disease organism may spread to the lungs or bloodstream and the central nervous system. The fatality rate when this happens is nearly 100%.

BLACK DEATH WAS NOT NECESSARILY BUBONIC PLAGUE

Not everyone believes that the bubonic plague organism caused the plague known as the Black Death. Two scientists from the Liverpool University School of Biological Sciences in England have published a book that places Europe's plague in a new historical, geographical, and demographic perspective. Using parish burial registers, Susan Scott and Christopher Duncan have shown that, although many of the symptoms match the bubonic plague, other factors, such as incubation times and transmission agents, do not. In their book, *The Biology of Plagues*, they show that the incubation period is too long and the type of rats most likely to carry the infected fleas

SIMOND SAYS

Dr. Paul-Louis Simond picked up plague research where Alexander Yersin left off. The prevailing sentiment of the day was that transmission of the plague was human-to-human. Yersin had hypothesized that rats were the main carriers. In spite of the prevailing wisdom, Simond began to uncover the evidence that would show that the fleas carried by rats were the main carriers of the disease. He developed a deceptively simple experiment that showed that the fleas killed the rat and then sought a new warm host—a human being. Simond published his work with the simple recommendation that the key to controlling plague was to keep rat populations in check. His work was met with silence or scorn. He remains a forgotten hero.

Source: Marriott, Edward. *Plague: A Story of Science, Rivalry, and the Scourge That Won't Go Away.* New York: Henry Holt and Company, LLC, 2003.

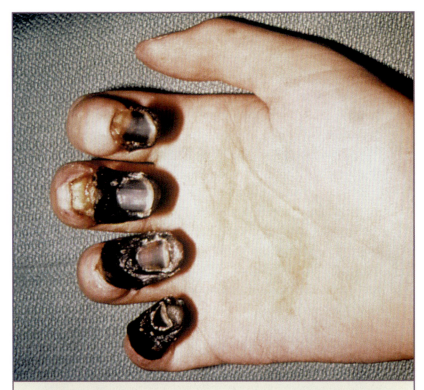

Figure 1.2 One possible effect of the plague is the development of gangrene. The plague bacterium, *Yersinia pestis*, most often causes blackened lumps called buboes (which led to the name "bubonic plague"). Gangrene is a similar symptom, in which the affected body part turns black because of insufficient blood flow. This person is suffering from gangrene on the hand. Gangrene is extremely dangerous because it can lead to the amputation of the rotted body part.

did not migrate into England until 50 years after the plague had ended in 1670. Quarantine measures are ineffective against bubonic plague, but they *were* successful against the Black Death. Scott and Duncan concluded after an exhaustive review of described symptoms and primitive autopsy results that the Black Death was probably caused by a virus distantly related to Ebola.

James Wood, professor of anthropology and demography at Penn State University, shares the opinion that bubonic plague was not the cause of the Black Death. Wood and several colleagues and graduate students have analyzed bishops' records of the replacement of priests during the time period of 1349–1350. From these records, Wood concluded that the disease spread much too rapidly among humans without being established in a wild rodent population first. Additionally, there were no records of widespread die-offs of rats in the streets or countryside. The disease spread rapidly along roadways and rivers, and was not slowed by the geographical barriers that normally would have stopped or restricted the movement of rodents. Wood and his colleagues have not ruled out the possibility that the causative agent might be an ancestor of the modern plague organism that mutated into the present form.

THE FRENCH AND ENGLISH CONTINUE TO DISAGREE

In another twist, researchers from Oxford University and Barts and London Hospital attempted to confirm reports of a French team that claimed to have isolated bits of *Yersinia pestis* DNA from the teeth of disinterred plague victims. The English team presented their results to the Society of General Microbiology at a conference in Manchester, England. They were unable to replicate the results of the French team. They found no *Yersinia pestis* DNA in any of the teeth of the victims they examined. They suggested that one future possibility would be to find a plague victim buried in the permafrost with enough preserved DNA to make a final determination.

Whether or not the Black Death and the bubonic plague are one and the same, the plague has caused enormous human devastation and has resulted in many changes in health and medical practices. The next few chapters will explore the cause of plague, the various forms that plague may take, the mechanisms of transmission, and the means available for prevention, treatment, and control of the disease. The final chapters look at our concerns and hopes for the future.

2

Causes of the Plague

Donner Memorial State Park near Truckee, California, closed on Tuesday, August 27, 2002. It would not reopen again until the spring of 2003. This would not seem to be a terribly unusual event except that the park normally stayed open for many more weeks. The immediate cause of this closing was confirmation of the plague in two squirrels, and the appearance of plague symptoms in a cat from a nearby park campground. Chipmunks and squirrels in the area had previously tested positive for the bubonic plague organism. "The Truckee area has a history of infected animals," said Vicki Kramer, chief of vector-borne diseases for the California health department.

ORIGIN OF THE PLAGUE ORGANISM

There are three human **pathogenic**, or disease-causing, species of the genus *Yersinia*: *Yersinia pestis*, which is the causative agent of the plague; *Yersinia pseudotuberculosis*; and *Yersinia enterocolitica*. The latter two species cause intestinal problems. *Y. enterocolitica* (for simplicity, genus names are often abbreviated), the most common of the three species and a very common form of food-borne sickness, causes **inflammation** of the intestines, a condition known as **gastroenteritis**. *Y. pseudotuberculosis*, the least common of the three, causes fever and abdominal pain that may mimic the symptoms of appendicitis.

Many scientists suggest that the bubonic plague organism has been around for millions of years. Dr. Victor Suntsov of the Severtsov Institute of Ecology and Evolution in the Russian Academy of Sciences suggests that the plague organism originated between 15,000 and 20,000 years ago in Mongolian marmots (small rodents similar to squirrels).

Suntsov contends that the plague microorganism evolved as a mutant form of *Yersinia pseudotuberculosis* in a population of marmots in Mongolia, Manchuria, and Transbailkal.

WHAT ARE BACTERIA?

Living things on this planet currently are placed into five large categories called kingdoms. These are the Plant Kingdom, Animal Kingdom, Fungi Kingdom, Protista Kingdom, and Bacteria (or Prokaryote) Kingdom.

The cells of all living organisms are organized in one of two ways. Cells from the Plant, Animal, Fungi, and Protista kingdoms all contain compartments constructed from internal cellular membranes. These compartments, which help separate chemicals and other materials from the interior of the cell, are called **organelles**, or miniature organs. Organelles include the nucleus, the lysosome, and the mitochondria. This type of cellular organization, with clearly defined and identifiable organelles, is described as the **eukaryotic** type of cellular organization. The term *eukaryotic* means "true nucleus" and comes from the Greek *eu*, meaning "true," and *karyon*, meaning "nucleus." Therefore, cells of plants, animals, fungi, and protozoa are known as eukaryotic cells, or eukaryotes, because of their internal cellular organization.

The Bacteria, or Prokaryote, Kingdom includes cells with a different type of internal organization. Bacterial cells lack membrane-defined organelles, are normally smaller than eukaryotic cells, and have few clearly defined internal structures. Because bacteria lack organelles such as the nucleus, they are described as being **prokaryotic** cells. The word *prokaryotic* comes from the Greek *pro*, for "before," and *karyon*, meaning "nucleus." Because bacterial cells do not have a nucleus, the genetic information (a single circular DNA molecule) resides in the cell with no membrane structure surrounding it. This type of cellular organization has served bacteria well for over 3.5 billion years.

IMPORTANT BACTERIAL STRUCTURES

Bacteria were originally classified as very small plants because, like plants, they have a cell wall protecting their cell membrane and the interior of the cell. However, bacterial cell walls are made of molecules that are different from the molecules in plant cell walls. Bacterial cell walls are made of a molecule called peptidoglycan that contains amino acids, which are building blocks made of proteins (*peptido*) and carbohydrates, which include simple sugars such as glucose (*glycan*). Because this unique molecule is not found among eukaryotes (including humans), the human immune system tries to remove or destroy it.

Bacteria have differing amounts of peptidoglycan in their cell walls. When treated with different dyes, these differences in the amount of peptidoglycan and other factors cause bacterial cells to retain or lose the color of specific dyes (Figure 2.1). One very famous and important staining reaction used to differentiate between bacteria is the Gram stain process. In

ARCHAEA—A THIRD FORM OF LIFE

Another group of microorganisms also has a prokaryotic type of cellular organization. They are called the archaebacteria, or simply the archaea, and they resemble bacteria in size and prokaryotic organization. However, the archaea are quite different genetically from both eukaryotic and prokaryotic types of cells. Archaea contain genetic information similar to the eukaryotes and also genetic information similar to bacteria. In addition, more than 40% of their genetic information is totally unique, resembling neither eukaryotes nor bacteria. The archaea live in extreme environments, earning them the name "extremophiles." Extreme environments include the absence of oxygen or places with very high heat, such as inside volcanoes.

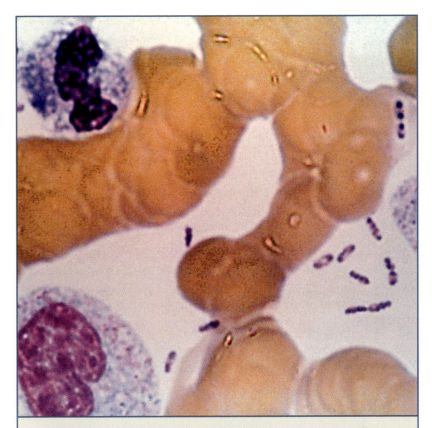

Figure 2.1 One way to test for the presence of the plague bacterium, *Yersinia pestis*, is with a procedure known as a Wright's stain, which takes a blood sample from a suspected plague patient and uses dye to detect bacteria in the blood. The darkened stains that indicate that the person has *Yersinia pestis* can be clearly seen on this sample of a Wright's stain.

this process, bacteria are treated with a series of different-colored dyes. If the bacteria retain the first dye color (crystal violet) throughout the entire staining procedure, they are called **gram-positive** bacteria. Other bacteria lose the first dye in the process and take on the color of the last dye (called the counterstain). These bacteria look pink or light red and are called **gram-negative** bacteria.

It is also important to know that bacteria can move on their own if they possess a structure called a flagellum (a whip-like tail). A **flagellum** (plural is *flagella*) helps the bacterium move toward areas where there is food and security and away from harmful areas. Flagella are made from a unique protein called **flagellin**. Because humans do not produce this protein, when the human immune system recognizes flagellin, it works to destroy it.

The unique molecular structure of bacterial cell walls and flagella is important to our understanding of the vaccines and drugs used against bubonic plague. For example, the unique structure of the peptidoglycan molecule makes it a target for antibiotics, such as penicillin, that have been very successful in killing the bacteria that cause many illnesses including bubonic plague.

CHARACTERISTICS OF *YERSINIA PESTIS*

Bacteria come in three basic shapes. A single bacterium shaped like a rod or a pencil is known as a **bacillus** (plural is *bacilli*). A bacterium shaped like a circle or a sphere is known as a **coccus** (plural is *cocci*). A bacterium that is shaped like a spiral or the letter "c," or is wound tightly like a spring, is known as a **spirillum** (plural is *spirilli*).

The bacterium responsible for bubonic plague is called *Yersinia pestis*. It is named after Alexander Yersin, who discovered it in 1894 while investigating the plague in Hong Kong. Yersin had originally named the organism *Pasteurella pestis* in honor of his mentor, Louis Pasteur. It is a small, stubby, gram-negative, oval- to rod-shaped bacterium. It is a **facultative anaerobe**, an organism that uses oxygen when it is present but can also live and reproduce in an **anaerobic** (oxygen-free) environment. *Yersinia pestis* tends to grow slowly in culture and produces small colonies.

When treated with certain dyes and staining techniques, *Yersinia pestis* creates an unusual staining pattern called

bipolar staining, which mimics a closed safety pin. Though this bipolar staining is not unique to *Yersinia pestis,* it is one of its many distinctive diagnostic characteristics.

FACTORS INVOLVED IN *YERSINIA*'S VIRULENCE

Yersinia pestis can multiply within a wide range of temperatures (-2°C to 45°C; 28.4°F to 113°F) and pH values (5.0 to 9.6), but optimal growth occurs at 28°C (82.4°F) and at a pH of about 7.4. The bacterium is **nonencapsulated**, or lacking a capsule or envelope, when it grows at its optimal growth temperature of 28°C. When grown at temperatures higher than 28°C, the organisms produce an envelope glycoprotein, called fraction 1 (F1). The genes for production of this glycoprotein are encoded in a **plasmid**. The F1 glycoprotein serves as an **antiphagocytic** capsule and allows the bacterium to obtain iron from its host. It also plays a role in the survival of the bacteria within the gut of a flea.

The bubonic plague organism, like other members of its family, the Enterobacteriaceae, is gram-negative. This is the same family that includes the common intestinal bacterium *Escherichia coli* and the *Salmonella* organisms, including the one that causes typhoid fever. The cell walls of gram-negative bacteria contain less peptidoglycan than those of gram-positive bacteria. The outermost layer of the cell wall of gram-negative bacteria also contains **lipopolysaccharide** (**LPS**) and proteins. Because LPS is toxic to mammals, it is called an **endotoxin**. When the bacterium dies, the LPS becomes free in the serum. Blood is divided into the formed elements (red and white blood cells and platelets) and the fluid portion, known as the plasma. When clotting factors, such as various proteins, are removed or neutralized, the light yellow fluid that is left is the serum. The serum contains the immune proteins known as antibodies; when free LPS interacts with these antibodies, a number of problems arise in humans, including fever, changing blood cell counts, and leaking blood vessels, which can lead to shock. This outer layer, also called the outer membrane, has an inside and an outside. The outside of the membrane contains the LPS. Part of this polysaccharide chain is a series of repeating sugar units known as O antigen. The name is derived from the fact that the polysaccharide is exposed to the outer environment. Host defenses can hone in on these sugars; however, bacteria can change the makeup of the O antigen to confuse the human host's immune system.

The outermost region of the cell wall is made of an inner phospholipid layer and an outer lipopolysaccharide layer. Just outside the cell membrane is a layer of peptidoglycan. Yersinia's cell wall is unlike that of other members of the Enterobacteriaceae family due to lack of O antigen side-chains. These O antigen side-chains are missing because a group of the bacteria's genes is disrupted.

The V (virulence) and W antigens are protein-lipoprotein complexes in the cell wall. These antigens make it difficult for white blood cells to engulf the bacteria. One important reason that Yersinia pestis is so virulent is its ability to survive and multiply within cells of the immune system. Antibodies produced against the V antigen provide protection against the plague organisms. Although it is not clear exactly how the V antigen works, it is obvious that it does multiple things. Any plague vaccine would include V antigen as an important component.

A protein called **invasin** on the outer membrane aids the bacterium in attachment to human cells. Another protein called plasminogen activator is an **enzyme** that aids in the spread of the bacteria. This enzyme prevents fibrin molecules from creating a clot formation that would trap the bacteria at the site of the fleabite.

NEEDLING THE HOST CELL

How do bacteria deliver toxins into a cell? The answer for a number of human pathogens, including Salmonella, Shigella, Chlamydia, Escherichia coli 0157:H7, and Yersinia, is a molecular

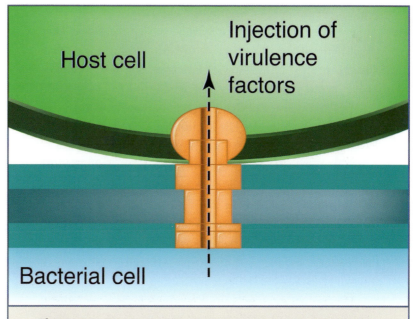

Figure 2.2 Plague has a unique way of injecting itself into a host cell. Once the bacterium's virulence genes have been activated, *Yersinia pestis* clamps on to a cell and acts almost like a syringe to force itself past the cell membrane. This process is sometimes referred to as "*Yersinia's* deadly kiss."

machine called the type III secretion system. The structure looks like a thumbtack or pushpin that you might put into a bulletin board (Figure 2.2).

This molecular machine is made of 29 proteins that, when assembled, "function as a syringe-like organelle spanning the cell membrane and anchored in the inner and outer membranes" of the cell wall. Dr. Susan Straley from the University of Kentucky explains how the needle-like molecular machine works: "When the needle—the part that sticks out—comes in contact with a host cell, it punctures the cell and samples the cytoplasm. In response to the low calcium environment inside the cell, the bug's [bacteria's] secretion mechanism is activated, and it sends toxins right into the host cytoplasm."

The toxins Straley mentioned are Yops (*Yersinia outer proteins*). Eleven of these proteins have been identified. They are structurally and functionally diverse, and include protein **kinases**, protein phosphatases, **proteases**, and **GAP proteins**. These proteins collectively overcome the host's natural defenses and make it difficult for the phagocytic white blood cells to become aware of the bacteria's presence. Once inside the host cell, they disrupt the **cytoskeleton** of the host cell, allowing the bacteria to multiply and spread within the host cell (Figure 2.3). "These Yops mimic key cell biological reactions and modify them in a way that is advantageous to the bacteria," Straley says. "One of the bug's early high-priority activities is to prevent being engulfed and destroyed by macrophages and PMNs (polymorphonucleated neutrophils); three of these Yops participate in that."

To summarize, the *Yersinia pestis* organism reproduces most rapidly at 27–28°C (80.6–82.4°F) but does not produce the protein toxins that are responsible for human symptoms at that temperature. When the microbe encounters a human cell with a temperature range of 36–38°C (96.8–100.4°F), its rate of reproduction slows but it begins to produce the apparatus needed to inject these proteins into its new human host. Also, at the higher temperatures, the microbes produce a capsule that makes it difficult for white blood cells to engulf them.

THE LIFE OF THE FLEA

Fleas survive best in a climate that is warm and moist (15–20°C [59–68°F] and 90–95% humidity). Changes in the seasons lead to temperature and humidity fluctuations that affect the life span and the level of activity of fleas. In most flea species, *Yersinia pestis* reproduces most rapidly at temperatures in the range of 26–28°C (78.8–82.4°F).

A flea acquires the disease by biting an infected host such as a rat or squirrel. After the microbe enters the flea's body, it reproduces rapidly and creates a plug of bacteria in the region

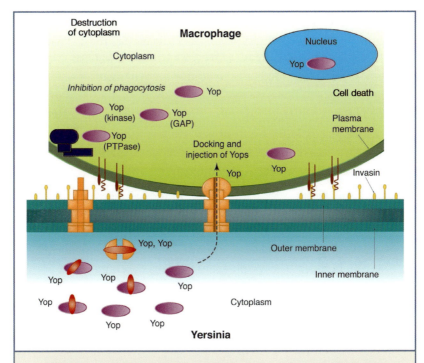

Figure 2.3 Once *Yersinia pestis* attaches, or "docks," onto a host cell, it causes infection by using Yops, or toxins, to inhibit the cell's normal functions. This diagram shows a *Yersinia* bacterium invading a macrophage, highlighting how the different Yops are injected into the host cell.

between the esophagus and the stomach. This plug prevents effective digestion by the flea. When the flea bites a human, the plug of bacteria is regurgitated into the new host's wound. The plague bacteria now begin to reproduce in the host's blood, causing the typical symptoms of plague and, often, the death of the host.

DIFFERENT MANIFESTATIONS OF THE PLAGUE

After the flea has found its new mammalian host, it takes a bite and injects some of the plague bacilli into the host's bloodstream. Some of the host's immune system cells—large, modified white blood cells called **macrophages**—are invaded by the plague organisms before the immune system recognizes the danger. Ironically, the bacteria find a safe place to live inside those cells whose job is supposed to be to destroy foreign organisms.

As the immune system becomes aware of the invasion, phagocytic white blood cells called polymorphonucleated neutrophils (PMNs) begin to gear up for action. The PMNs destroy many of the bacteria but are overwhelmed by the sheer numbers of the microbes. Additionally, the microbes begin to produce capsules and other proteins that prevent destruction by the PMNs. At this point, the microbes may enter the **lymphatic system**. This fluid-filled system runs parallel to the circulatory system and has a series of collection regions known as **lymph nodes**. The lymph nodes have large accumulations of PMNs, macrophages, and other chemical agents. The bacteria that enter the lymphatic system are filtered through the lymph nodes, and a battle is joined between the bacteria and the immune system cells and chemicals. This battle causes an inflammatory reaction that signals additional cells to join the fight. It also results in a swollen lymph node known as a **bubo**. This feature is diagnostic of the bubonic form of the plague. It usually takes from 2 to 7 days for a swollen lymph node to develop after the fleabite. The lymph carries the bacteria back into the bloodstream, where they enter the liver and the spleen. While many bacteria are undoubtedly killed by immune system cells in these organs, their sheer number tends to overwhelm the body's defenses.

Some bacteria wind up in the lungs, producing a highly contagious and extremely dangerous form of plague. Known as **pneumonic** plague, the bacteria can be spread from person to person by coughing. According to Dr. Susan Straley, inhaling as few as 100 of the bacteria can cause pneumonic plague. Given the fact that scientists estimate each square centimeter of our skin holds an average of 100,000 bacteria, these 100 bugs pack an extraordinary punch.

Because the inhaled bacteria have already adapted to the body of the first person, they arrive fully armed with their toxin-delivery mechanism. Straley says this gives the bacteria a head start in the race against the body's defenses. As in bubonic plague, the bacteria first encounter macrophages—in this case, alveolar macrophages, the lungs' defense cells. "Some of the bacteria go into macrophages, you get an influx of PMNs and then inflammation. Part of inflammation is fluid influx, so your lungs fill up and you can't breathe," says Straley. "The bacteria also spread to the lymph nodes and the blood, so the basic process is the same as in bubonic plague, but we really know very little about the specifics. As little as one day after inhalation you start showing severe symptoms of pneumonia, and the next day you could be dead." Straley adds that this is a very narrow window for correct diagnosis and treatment.

Septicemic plague may occur as a complication of either bubonic or pneumonic plague. It is not spread from person to person but is characterized by the presence of bacteria in the bloodstream. Of the three forms, pneumonic plague is the most deadly and the fastest killer.

3

Cats, Rats, Prairie Dogs, and Squirrels

Jim was about to get his airline tickets online. He had been fortunate to get a good rate for the trip to Albuquerque, New Mexico. His university's spring break was a little later than many others were, so he wouldn't get involved with all the usual traffic. It also helped that most people headed south to Florida or the Caribbean on spring break. Jim was going to spend a few days with a friend he had met in India that previous summer. Jim had been in New Delhi at the All India Institute as part of a program to learn about the health-care system of a large urban city. A select group of American university students had been chosen to observe and, when possible, work with the staff and doctors at the Institute.

THE VISIT

One of the students who had also been in India with Jim was a young man by the name of Zachary Nisrey. From the first day they met, Jim knew that Zachary was a person with whom he wanted to spend some time. Zachary was extremely bright and soft-spoken. He listened intently to everything the doctors and staff had to say and picked up the Institute routines quickly. But Zachary also had a devilish side, which he showed with a variety of practical jokes. Always clever but never harmful or nasty, it seemed that Zachary knew how to make people laugh. When their time in India ended, the new friends exchanged e-mail addresses and promised to visit each other. Eight months later, a visit would take place.

Zachary lived south of Santa Fe, about 25 miles (40 km) away from Albuquerque. He was a student at the University of New Mexico in

Albuquerque, enrolled in the department of Family and Community Medicine. Jim was enrolled in the department of Health Science Administration in the College of Health Sciences at his local university, so there was considerable overlap in their college backgrounds.

Mid-April in Albuquerque and Santa Fe meant high temperatures ranging between 60 and 70°F (15.6–21.1°C) and low temperatures between 35 and 45°F (1.7–7.2°C). The previous year had been wetter than normal, but no rain appeared to be scheduled for the week of Jim's trip. Jim thought about what he would need to pack for the range of temperatures and for activities that would range from mountain hiking to walking through the desert. He was happy he didn't have to get all the vaccinations that had been required for his India trip the previous summer. Zachary had promised to pick up Jim from the airport and give him a quick tour of the university campus before they headed home. Jim was counting the days until the beginning of the spring break and the trip to New Mexico.

FIRST STOP—THE HOSPITAL?

Jim's flight to Albuquerque was uneventful. When Jim stepped off the plane, Zachary was waiting to greet him. Grinning widely, Zachary shook Jim's hand firmly. "Great to see you again," he said. After collecting Jim's luggage, they got into Zachary's car and headed out of the airport. "The university is along the way, so we'll stop there and you'll also get a chance to meet my dad," proclaimed Zachary.

"That's great," said Jim. "Does your father work at the university?" asked Jim.

"No," said Zachary, "he's in the university hospital."

"What's wrong with him?" asked Jim, hoping he had not made the trip at the wrong time.

"He's got bubonic plague," stated Zachary, showing little emotion in his voice.

"BUBONIC PLAGUE!" shouted Jim. There was what seemed to be a long silence before Zachary replied. In actuality, it was less than ten seconds. A smile crossed Zachary's face as they entered the university grounds. For a moment, Jim thought this might have been another of Zachary's practical jokes.

"Apparently you didn't do your homework before you came to this area of New Mexico," said Zachary. "If you had, you would have known that New Mexico has an average of 7 to 8 cases of plague each year. The Santa Fe area has become somewhat famous in the last few years for plague cases. Have you heard of John Tull and Lucinda Marker?" asked Zachary.

"Can't say that I have," replied Jim.

Zachary continued: "They are a married couple who became infected by the plague organism from the fleas of a dead rat on their property near Santa Fe. They went to New York for a vacation and wound up in the hospital there. Caused quite a stir at the hospital, since none of the doctors had ever seen a plague case before and now they had two patients at once. John was in bad shape and spent a long time recovering. As a matter of fact, he only took his first steps without a walker back on December 1, 2003."

Zachary explained that John became so ill that the doctors had to amputate both of his legs below the knee, and that there is a Web site (*http://www.johnandlucinda.com*) that allows viewers to keep track of how John is doing.

Zachary's car pulled up next to a building with a sign that said Health Sciences Center. "Here's where I spend most of my time on campus. We can walk over to the university hospital after I take you on a quick tour of the facilities." Jim was happy to get out and stretch his legs again, but he was flabbergasted at this turn of events. He had never seen a person who had bubonic plague. If he remembered his microbiology correctly, the plague was also called the Black Death. What would Zachary's father look like? Would his extremities be all black and gangrenous? Zachary didn't seem that concerned. As a matter of fact, Zachary appeared to be no more concerned than if his father had contracted a cold. It was time to go see Zachary's father over at the hospital. As they walked, Zachary explained how his father had contracted the disease.

WEEKEND AT CAMP

Three weeks ago, Zachary's father, Al Nisrey, visited a friend in an area near Bluewater Lake in northwestern New Mexico, not far from Albuquerque. They were going to do some repairs on the friend's hunting cabin. Rodents had gnawed through some of the wooden planks, and the cabin was open to the environment. Among the unwanted guests in the cabin were a number of dead rock squirrels. Since it had been a tough winter, the dead squirrels did not seem unusual. Al and his friend used gloves and carefully removed the squirrels and burned their bodies in a large bonfire. They noticed that the squirrels had acquired large numbers of fleas. Some had crawled onto Al's arms and bitten him. His friend also was bitten by the fleas. They used a pesticide spray to kill the fleas. Unfortunately for them, the damage had already been done.

After a weekend of repair work on the cabin, Al headed for home. He was beginning to feel like he was coming down with the flu. His throat was sore, his body ached, and he felt alternately feverish and then chilled. He would have dismissed all of these symptoms except for the fact that he was starting to feel weak and had itchy fleabites on his arms and legs. The regional lymph nodes under his arms and in his groin region were swollen and tender to the touch. Al called home on his cell phone and spoke to Zachary. He told Zachary he was going directly to the hospital and would call after he had checked in. Al Nisrey had lived in New Mexico long enough to know that symptoms like his could easily mean bubonic plague. His friend joined him in the hospital the following day.

Al Nisrey had indeed contracted bubonic plague. His fast action in going to the hospital had saved his family from having to take antibiotics. If he had come home and interacted with the family, all of the members would have to take antibiotics as a precaution against contracting the disease.

As Zachary and Jim got to his room, Al Nisrey greeted a somewhat hesitant Jim with a big smile and the reassurance that he was not contagious. Al was responding nicely to the antibiotic therapy and was looking quite well. He would soon be coming home. If Jim had not known of the illness, he would never have guessed that Al had bubonic plague. He now understood why Zachary did not appear to be concerned about his father's health.

WHAT TYPES OF ANIMALS CARRY THE PLAGUE ORGANISM?

As is true with many diseases, humans are not the primary host of the disease organism *Yersinia pestis*. Human infection is accidental or incidental, and depends on the chance contact between humans and the infected fleas of infected rodents (Figure 3.1). In other words, Zachary's dad was in the wrong place at the wrong time. Animal hosts, such as the rock squirrels, will usually begin to die off in increasing numbers before humans are likely to be infected, because the fleas of the dying rodents will be seeking new hosts. Zachary's dad did not see or recognize the increase in the number of dead squirrels. He only saw the dead squirrels in the cabin.

DIFFERENT LEVELS OF INFECTION

Some animal groups are fairly resistant to the impact of the plague organisms. Mice of the genus *Microtus* or the genus *Peromyscus* are considered **enzootic reservoirs** of the infection. This means that the frequency of the plague organism is maintained at a low level in the population of host organisms (the mice), resulting in low mortality rates. This difference in resistance to the plague organism varies from one geographical region to another.

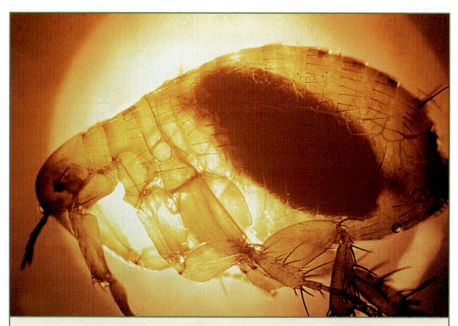

Figure 3.1 Plague is spread through the bite of infected fleas, which acquire the bacterium from rats and other rodents that are known carriers of *Yersinia pestis*. This is an oriental rat flea, or *Xenopsylla cheopis*. The dark mass in its lower body, which scientists call a proventricular plague mass, is evidence that the flea is infected with plague.

In contrast, there are a number of animal species that are highly susceptible to the *Yersinia pestis* organism. These species seem to be clustered in the western part of the United States and represent the greatest threat to the human population. The hosts are mostly rodents that die in large numbers, causing the fleas to change hosts. This group of highly susceptible animals is called an **epizootic reservoir**. Included in this group are urban and domestic rats, ground squirrels, rock squirrels, prairie dogs, gerbils, voles, chipmunks, marmots, guinea pigs, and kangaroo rats.

Although rodents get most of the blame, mammals can also introduce infected fleas to humans or to other animal species.

SYLVATIC AND URBAN PLAGUE

When plague organisms are found mainly in the fleas of rodents, such as squirrels, in areas away from where humans live, the disease is called **sylvatic plague**. Infection is accidental and incidental, and is usually not the cause of epidemics. When plague organisms are found in the fleas of rats in and around densely populated cities, the disease is called **urban plague**. This kind of plague has traditionally been the cause of epidemics (Figure 3.2).

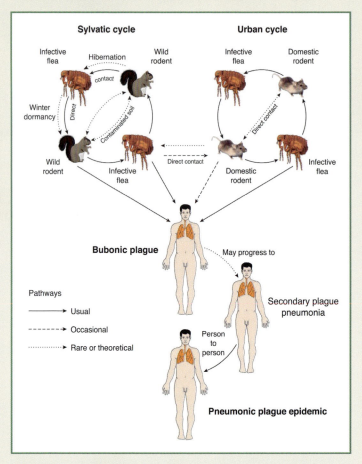

Figure 3.2 Although humans most often get plague from the bite of an infected flea, this diagram shows some of the other possible ways to catch the disease.

Coyotes, badgers, rabbits and hares, deer, antelope, goats, camels, cats, and sometimes dogs can all transmit the fleas to human beings. As humans and their animal pets continue to expand their living quarters into the habitats of wild mammals and rodents, increased contact is inevitable. With this increased contact comes the likelihood of transmitting disease organisms between species.

4

Diagnosis

About twenty minutes after leaving the hospital, Zachary pulled into the driveway of his home. Zachary's brother Garrett greeted them. "Dad called and said you were on the way and that Jim had arrived on time," said Garrett. "I made some coffee and Mom said you could have some of the cake in the refrigerator. She'll be home in about an hour." Zachary thanked his brother as he poured a cup of coffee for himself and one for Jim. After bringing in Jim's luggage and getting him settled in the guest room, the two young men sat out on the back porch and enjoyed the warmth of the coffee and the crispness of the fresh air.

"You wanted to know how they figured out that my dad really had the plague. You asked the right person, so sit back and I'll give you an overview of what happens," said Zachary. Trying to diagnose a disease strictly on the basis of its symptoms is not very useful, Zachary explained, since many diseases have similar symptoms. Everything from the flu to various types of food poisoning may have symptoms including headache, fever, chills, body aches, and overall weakness. Diagnosis of bubonic plague requires that health-care workers carry out laboratory tests on the patient's blood, sputum (material coughed up from the lungs), or the fluid taken from an enlarged or swollen lymph node (a bubo). Suspected plague organisms can be stained using a Gram stain or Wayson's stain. Usually, a chest X-ray is taken to determine whether the plague organism has entered the lungs. Diagnosis of the different forms of the plague involves modifications of some of the techniques.

FORMS OF THE PLAGUE

The same bacterium can cause three different forms of plague. The bubonic form is best known because of the swollen and tender lymph nodes called buboes. If the organisms invade the bloodstream, they may cause destruction of blood vessels under the skin, leading to the darkened or blackened areas that gave the Black Death its name. Usually, the patient's high fever, over 104°F, leads to delirium and, in more than half of all untreated cases, death.

The bacterium may invade the lungs and cause a pneumonic form of the disease. This form is extremely contagious and is the most dangerous form, since it is spread from person to person through aerosol droplets. Every time the patient coughs or sneezes, he or she may contaminate people in the area. Victims of this form of plague usually develop a severe cough and eventually bloody sputum. Pneumonic plague leads to coma and death in nearly 100% of untreated cases.

The third form of plague occurs when large numbers of the bacteria enter the bloodstream. This is known as the septicemic form. It normally causes gangrene in various body areas, and death usually occurs within a day or two. Untreated, all infected people die from this form of plague.

DIAGNOSIS OF BUBONIC PLAGUE

The incubation period for the bubonic form of the plague ranges from 2 to 10 days. Patients are often tired, have a fever as high as 105°F (40.6°C), and exhibit tender lymph nodes, particularly in the groin region or areas near the fleabite. The liver and spleen may also be tender. About one-fourth of all bubonic plague patients may have skin lesions. A presumptive diagnosis is usually made microscopically when gram-negative coccobacillary cells show a "safety pin" or bipolar staining pattern. This staining pattern is the result of granules that are localized in the ends of the cell. The sample may be taken from a lymph node, sputum, or cerebrospinal fluid. If it is available, immunofluorescent staining can also provide useful information.

A definitive diagnosis is made when the organisms are cultured on various microbiological media such as blood agar, MacConkey agar, or infusion broth. *Y. pestis* does not have many enzymatic functions, such as adenine deaminase, aspartase, ornithine decarboxylase, glucose-6-phosphate dehydrogenase, and urease. It primarily utilizes glucose and mannitol, and cannot ferment most carbohydrates. It grows on sheep blood agar with little or no hemolysis, and forms gray-white colonies with a shiny appearance after about 48 hours. The colony borders are irregular, and are often termed "fried-egg." Positive cultures that display the above characteristics are considered evidence of *Y. pestis* infection, and are reported and forwarded, if necessary, to state authorities for further identification and confirmation.

LABORATORY DIAGNOSIS AND SAFETY

Microscopic examination of stained samples from body fluids and the use of immunofluorescent stains provide the first evidence of the possibility of *Yersinia pestis* infection. The diagnosis is confirmed through **serology**, in which characteristics of a disease are shown through the study of blood serums, but because *Yersinia pestis* is a slow grower and takes about two days to grow on blood or MacConkey agar, serology is not useful if a rapid diagnosis is needed. If antibodies against the bacterial capsule (F1 antigen) are found to have increased at least fourfold in a patient with no history of plague vaccination, then this confirms the original diagnosis.

HANDLING LABORATORY SPECIMENS

Laboratory work on those suspected of having *Y. pestis* infection should be done in Biosafety Level 2 facilities, using

SUMMARY OF LABORATORY DIAGNOSIS FOR SUSPECTED PLAGUE CASES

STAINING OF SPECIMENS

- **Appropriate clinical specimens include**: Blood, bubo aspirates, sputum, cerebrospinal fluid (CSF) (if there are signs/symptoms of meningitis), and skin scrapings (if a lesion is present).

- **Gram stain**: Polymorphonuclear leukocytes and bipolar staining, "safety-pin" ovoid, gram-negative cocco-bacilli identified in bubo aspirate, sputum, or CSF are highly suggestive of plague.

- **Wayson stain**: *Yersinia pestis* appears as light blue bacilli with dark blue polar bodies on a contrasting pink ground.

- **Immunofluorescent staining of capsule (F1)**: A positive finding is diagnostic. Must use fresh specimens to avoid false negatives. This test is available only at reference laboratories.

BACTERIAL CULTURES

- Blood, bubo aspirates, sputum, CSF, and skin scrapings can be cultured.

- Materials should be inoculated into blood and MacConkey agar plates and infusion broth. It generally takes 2 days to identify visible colonies. Rapid biochemical identification systems may not be reliable for identification due to slower growth rate of *Y. pestis*.

SEROLOGIC TESTING

- Several serologic tests are available, including a passive hemagglutination test (CDC). A fourfold or greater rise is diagnostic, a single titer (concentration) of >1:16 in someone without prior immunization against plague is suggestive. Serology is not useful for rapid diagnosis.

Source: Medical Treatment and Response to Suspected Plague: Information for Health Care Providers During Biologic Emergencies, New York City Department of Health, Bureau of Communicable Disease. Available online at *http://www.nyc.gov/html/doh/html/cd/plaguemd.html#five*.

standard and special practices, equipment, and facility specifications. For example, staff must wear surgical gloves, protective gowns, and shoe covers. Staff must make every effort to avoid splashing or creating an aerosol, and must wear protective eyewear and masks if work cannot be done in a Biosafety Level 2 cabinet.

Yersinia pestis is classified as a select agent, one with the potential to pose a severe threat to public health and safety, and, therefore, its handling is regulated under strict federal guidelines. These provide requirements for laboratories that handle select agents such as *Y. pestis,* including registration, security risk assessments, safety plans, security plans, emergency response plans, training, transfers, record keeping, inspections, and notifications. The requirements went into effect on February 7, 2003. They supersede earlier government requirements for the handling and transfer of particular agents.

LEVELS OF LABORATORY ACTIVITIES

Laboratories are categorized into four levels: A, B, C, and D. Level A laboratories can perform the standard initial tests designed to rule out (but not definitively identify) *Y. pestis.* They include Clinical Laboratory Improvement Act (CLIA)–certified clinical laboratories with Biosafety Level 2 (BSL-2) equipment and practices. The protocols for Level A laboratories include Gram stains, spot tests, and other simple tests such as motility tests. The intent is to rule out agents of bioterrorism.

Level B laboratories have the ability and capacity for agent isolation and confirmatory testing and include most state public health laboratories. Level B laboratories are expected to perform biochemical identification of *Brucella, Francisella, Yersinia,* and *Bacillus* species to rule out agents of bioterrorism. They require a minimum of BSL-2 and usually BSL-3. Level C laboratories have advanced capacity for rapid identification and include selected public health, federal, and

SUMMARY OF RECOMMENDED BIOSAFETY LEVELS (BSL) FOR INFECTIOUS AGENTS

BSL	Agents	Practices	Safety Equipment (Primary Barriers)	Facilities (Secondary Barriers)
1	Not known to cause disease in healthy adults	Standard microbiological practices	Not required	Open bench top sink required
2	Associated with human disease; hazard: auto-inoculation, ingestion, mucous membrane exposure	BSL-1 practice plus: limited access, biohazard warning signs, "Sharps" precautions, biosafety manual defining any needed waste decontamination or medical surveillance policies	Primary barriers: Class I or II BSCs* or other physical containment devices used for all manipulations of agents that cause splashes or aerosols of infectious materials; PPEs*: laboratory coats, gloves, face protection as needed	BSL-1 plus: autoclave available
3	Indigenous or exotic agents with potential for aerosol transmission; disease may have serious or lethal consequences	BSL-2 practice plus: controlled access, decontamination of lab clothing before laundering, baseline serum	Primary barriers: Class I or II BSCs or other physical containment devices used for all manipulations of agents; PPEs: protective lab clothing, gloves, respiratory protection is needed	BSL-2 plus: physical separation from access corridors; self-closing, double door access; exhausted exhausted air not recirculated; negative airflow into laboratory
4	Dangerous/exotic agents that pose high risk of life-threatening disease, aerosol-transmitted lab infections, or related agents with unknown risk of transmission	BSL-3 practice plus: clothing change before entering, shower on exit, all material decontaminated on exit from facility	Primary barriers: all procedures conducted in Class III BSCs or Class I or II BSCs in combination with full-body, air-supplied, positive pressure personnel suit	BSL-3 plus: separate building, or isolated zone, dedicated supply/ exhaust, vacuum, and decon systems, other requirements outlined in the text

* BSCs = Biosafety cabinets
* PPEs = Personal protection equipment

View the entire CDC/NIH Biosafety Guidelines online at
http://www.research.umich.edu/policies/um/committees/BRRC/BSLChartCDCNIH.html.

THE LABORATORY RESPONSE NETWORK (LRN)

The Laboratory Response Network (LRN) is a network of laboratories that have been developed to coordinate all clinical diagnostic testing for suspected bioterrorism events. The network was established in 1999 and consists of public health laboratories that form links with private hospital, clinical, and referral labs that normally send suspected select agents to the public health labs for confirmation of the suspected organism. The LRN categorizes laboratories into four levels, based on their capabilities, with Level A at the base and Level D at the top (Figure 4.1).

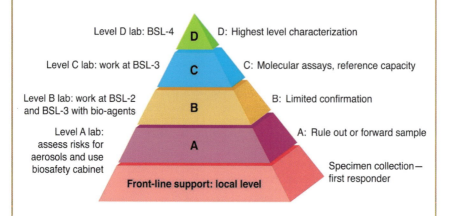

Level D lab: BSL-4 — D: Highest level characterization

Level C lab: work at BSL-3 — C: Molecular assays, reference capacity

Level B lab: work at BSL-2 and BSL-3 with bio-agents — B: Limited confirmation

Level A lab: assess risks for aerosols and use biosafety cabinet — A: Rule out or forward sample

Specimen collection— first responder

Front-line support: local level

Figure 4.1 In the post-9/11 world, the fear of biological terror attacks is widespread. To help prevent the possible spread of dangerous diseases, like plague, that might be used as weapons, a complex system called the Laboratory Response Network has been set up to track the course of plague and other illnesses in unusual situations. From the initial report of the disease, the conditions and risks are assessed by more and more specialized laboratories until the situation is firmly understood and under control.

academic laboratories. They require BSL-4 safety equipment and practices.

Level D laboratories have the highest level of containment (BSL-4) and expertise in the diagnosis of rare and dangerous biological agents, and include specialized federal laboratories. Specific information about Level B, C, and D protocols for *Y. pestis* is not available to the public.

5
Treatment

After dinner with Zachary's family, Jim and Zachary sat down with another cup of coffee and talked more about the plague.

Zachary said, "It's really amazing when you consider that an average of only 10 *Yersinia pestis* microorganisms need to invade the body in order to cause bubonic plague. But it's equally amazing to me that our bodies use secretions of other bacteria to kill off the first bacteria. I know that this is a natural series of events that has been occurring for millions of years. This competition has helped to maintain a balance between microbes and larger organisms like humans. It's hard to believe that until less than a century ago, we had few ways to aid us in the fight against bacterial diseases. You tend to take antibiotics for granted until they are needed to cure someone close to you."

EARLY TREATMENTS FOR THE PLAGUE

Since their discovery and development in the 1940s, **antibiotics** have taken the lead in fighting the effects of bacterial diseases. Prior to the use of antibiotics, however, people employed a number of unique and unusual treatments. Some, such as the use of garlic and silver compounds to ward off infection by bacteria, were based on folk medicine passed down through generations. Others, such as trying to purify the air with rosemary and thyme, were based on uncritical human observations that sometimes led to false conclusions.

Before the discovery and study of microorganisms such as bacteria, European medical thought was dominated by what an Italian historian named Carlo Cipolla has called the "miasmatic paradigm." (*Miasma* refers to a thick, vaporous atmosphere.) Contagion was thought to arise from exposure to unhealthy, "corrupted" air, although the exact nature of this dangerous influence was unspecified.

In Seville, Spain, in the 1600s, city officials made residents clean the streets, burn the clothing and bedding of the sick, and isolate people who were clearly ill. The officials recommended that people add rosemary and thyme to the air for the purpose of purification. Variants of these techniques continue to be used today in some disease settings; for example, the burning corresponds to sterilization of materials, and isolation of people with disease is obviously a method of quarantine.

In today's world, we know that disease transmission and prevention is related to sanitary conditions. A clean environment reduces the likelihood of disease organisms being spread from animals to people and between people. That is why some of the early treatments for the plague, such as bathing in human urine, wearing human excrement, and placing dead animals in homes (called "stinks"), seem so strange to us. The use of leeches (a worm-like animal that sucks blood) was a common mechanism for treating many illnesses. Drinking molten gold (gold heated until it melted) and powdered emeralds was also recommended but was usually fatal. Some suggestions, such as eating figs before 6:00 A.M., chopping up a snake every day, falling asleep on the left side of the bed, or not sleeping during the day, make no obvious medical sense and seem to be home-remedy suggestions.

People from all lifestyles sought ways to protect themselves from disease. Grave robbers used garlic to protect against bubonic plague by washing themselves, their clothes, and stolen items with garlic vinegar. French priests of the Middle Ages used garlic as well as prayer to protect themselves against bubonic plague (Figure 5.1).

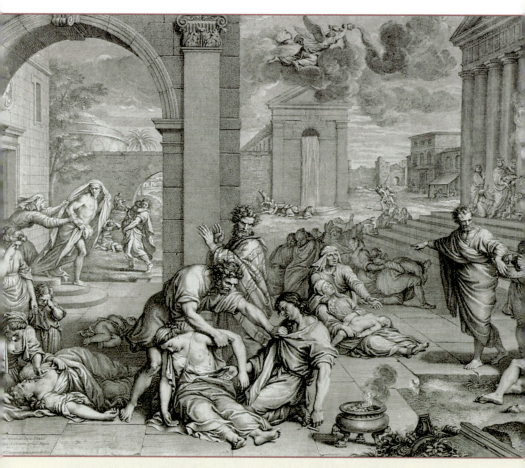

Figure 5.1 During the Middle Ages (between about A.D. 500 and 1500), the plague was a terrible threat to humans. It killed vast numbers of people and devastated the population of Europe. Those who could afford to do so often fled cities during warmer weather, which was considered "plague season." This illustration by C. Audran, done in the 17th century, depicts the chaos and horrible suffering that resulted from an outbreak of plague.

CURRENT TREATMENT

When left untreated, plague can result in rapid death. Approximately 14 to 17% of all plague cases in the United States each year are fatal. However, if treatment is received early enough, five out of six patients survive. "My father increased his chance of survival by going directly to the hospital," said Zachary. He informed the hospital admissions personnel that he thought he had bubonic plague because of his symptoms and his contact with fleas. Because plague was suspected, Al Nisrey was immediately isolated and local and state departments were notified. Antibiotic treatment reduces the risk of death to less than 5%. Streptomycin is the preferred treatment and should be given immediately upon admission to the hospital. Other possible useful antibiotics include gentamicin, chloramphenicol, tetracycline, and trimethoprim-sulfamethoxazole.

The patient's own doctor will determine the specific treatment for plague based on a number of factors, including the patient's age, overall health, and medical history. The patient's ability to tolerate specific medications, procedures, or therapies will also be considered. In each case, the patient will be hospitalized and medically isolated and given immediate antibiotic treatment. The isolation continues for 48 hours after antibiotic therapy is begun or until cultures are negative. Gloves are worn at all times when in contact with the infected individual and hospital personnel must avoid contact with all bodily fluids (urine, sputum, saliva, blood, and semen). If plague bacteria are found in a blood smear, they indicate septicemic plague.

TREATMENT OF PNEUMONIC PLAGUE

Treatment for the pneumonic form of plague is different from other forms because it can be spread from person to person by droplet transmission (i.e., coughing and sneezing). When caring for patients with suspected or confirmed plague, hospital personnel must be especially cautious. Patients with pneumonic plague should be placed on strict respiratory isolation until appropriate antibiotics have been administered for 48 hours and the patient shows clinical improvement. Droplet precautions require that the patient be placed in a private room and that anyone entering the patient's room must wear a surgical mask, particularly when standing within 3 feet (1 meter) of the patient. Because transmission can occur from plague skin lesions (such as draining buboes or abscesses) to contacts, if such skin lesions are present, wound and skin precautions should be followed. Traditionally, streptomycin, tetracycline, and doxycycline have been used for the treatment of plague and are approved by the Food and Drug Administration (FDA) for this indication. Rifampin, aztreonam, ceftazidime, cefotetan, and cefazolin have been shown to be ineffective and should not be used to treat plague. The Working Group on Civilian Biodefense also developed consensus-based recommendations for treatment of pneumonic plague during a bioterrorist attack. The Working Group made the recommendations outlined in Table 5.1.

If a person becomes exposed to airborne or aerosolized *Yersinia pestis* or comes into close physical contact with a patient who has a confirmed case of pneumonic plague, he or she must receive antibiotic therapy. Individuals to whom this precaution applies would include people in the same household and health-care workers. All antibiotic therapy should continue for seven days from the date of the *last exposure* to the organism or infected patient.

TREATING ENVIRONMENTAL SURFACES

Since September 11, 2001, governmental officials have been concerned about the possible use of bacteria such as anthrax and plague as biological weapons by terrorists. Law enforcement officials have the right to test for the presence of these organisms if it is suspected that an environmental surface has been contaminated. Jim and the Nisrey family would be in minimal danger, since *Yersinia pestis* is not known to remain viable for very long periods on most external surfaces. Some surfaces, however, are an exception. Cells of

Table 5.1 Recommendations from the Working Group on Civilian Biodefense for Treatment of Pneumonic Plague During a Bioterroism Event

Patient Category	Recommended Therapy
	Contained Casualty Setting
Adults	**Prefererred choices**
	Streptomycin, 1 g IM 2 times daily for 10 days*
	Gentamicin, 5 mg/kg IM or IV once daily or 2 mg/kg loading dose followed by 1.7 mg/kg IM or IV 3 times daily
	Alternative choices
	Doxycycline, 100 mg IV 2 times daily or 200 mg IV once daily
	Ciprofloxacin, 400 mg IV 2 times daily
	Chloramphenicol, 25 mg/kg IV 4 times daily
Children	**Prefererred choices**
	Streptomycin, 15 mg IM 2 times daily (maximum daily dose, 2 g)
	Gentamicin, 2.5 mg/kg IM or IV 3 times daily
	Alternative choices
	Doxycycline
	If ≥45 kg, give adult dosage
	If <45 kg, give 2.2 mg/kg IV 2 times daily (maximum, 200 mg/day)
	Ciprofloxacin, 15 mg/kg IV 2 times daily
	Chloramphenicol, 25 mg/kg IV 4 times daily
Pregnant women	**Prefererred choices**
	Gentamicin, 5 mg/kg IM or IV once daily or 2 mg/kg loading dose followed by 1.7 mg/kg IM or IV 3 times daily
	Alternative choices
	Doxycycline, 100 mg IV 2 times daily or 200 mg IV once daily
	Ciprofloxacin, 400 mg IV 2 times daily

* All recommended therapies should last 10 days unless otherwise noted.

Recommended Antibiotics
The drug of choice for primary pneumonic plague is streptomycin administered by intramuscular injection every 12 hours for 10 days. However, since streptomycin may be in short supply, gentamicin administered every 8 hours intravenously or intramuscularly for 10 days and doxycycline followed by 100 mg IV every 12 hours for 10–14 days, are alternative agents. Chloramphenicol should be used for plague meningitis due to its better central nervous system (CNS) penetration.

Antibiotic choice may need to be altered as susceptibility information becomes available.

Alternative Antibiotics
Ciprofloxacin, levofloxacin, and ofloxacin are acceptable alternative agents. The efficacy of quinolones in humans has not been formally evaluated.

Bactrim may also be useful based on animal and *in vitro* studies.

Much less effective drugs (do not use unless all other alternatives are unavailable) include: rifampin, aztreonam, ampicillin, ceftazadime, cefotetan and cefazolin.

Supportive Therapy
Supportive care is essential, including intravenous fluids and monitoring of changes in the bloodstream volume and contents.

Therapy in pediatric patients, in newborns up to age 2 months, and in pregnant women must be monitored and treated differently from a normal patient.

Source: From information available online at *http://www.nyc.gov/html/doh/html/cd/plaguemd.html#five.*

NONTOXIC DISINFECTANT KILLS BUBONIC PLAGUE

American Biotech Labs has a disinfectant called ASAP-AGX-32 that has been approved by the Environmental Protection Agency (EPA) for use against gram-negative bacteria, including *Yersinia pestis*. The company was interested in determining how well the disinfectant would actually work on *Y. pestis*. It did its work at a Biosafety Level 3 (BSL-3) laboratory, testing the disinfectant against a concentration of 81 million bacteria per milliliter (ml), a dose that is 160 times greater than the 500,000 per ml that is the normal *in vitro* (performed in a test tube) test dosage. Even at this higher bacterial load, all bacteria were killed in less than 2 minutes. "The ASAP-AGX-32 (EPA registration No. 73499-2) product has already been approved by the EPA for use against gram-negative bacteria, and *Y. pestis* is a gram-negative bacterium," said Keith Moeller, vice president of American Biotech Labs. "We wanted to test the limits of the product's capability, and we are delighted with the results."

Another unique aspect of the disinfectant is that it is odorless and colorless. "Unlike other disinfectants, the ASAP-AGX-32 can be used or sprayed around both adults and children with no toxic effect. The product is not known to irritate the skin, eyes, nose, or lungs," noted Moeller.

It would seem that this product may prove to be very useful in a variety of medical and industrial settings. "To date, this product has killed every strain of every bacterium on which it has been tested. It has received EPA approval for use against the most deadly bacteria, including gram-negative, gram-positive and even nosocomial or hospital acquired (superbug) pathogens. The product has been approved for use as a broad spectrum, general use surface disinfectant in homes, hospitals, and medical settings," said Moeller.

Source: Available online at *http://www.hartamerica.com/ASAP-AGX-32.htm*.

Yersinia pestis have been shown to live up to 6 hours on steel, 7 hours on glass, 24 hours on polyethylene, and 120 hours on paper. Very few commercial chemicals have been marketed specifically for destruction of this organism. These types of samples must be tested at a Level B or higher LRN laboratory.

6

Prevention

There are a number of basic, commonsense methods that can be effective in the prevention of the plague. In addition, vaccination or prophylactic use of antibiotics is advised for people who may be exposed to the fleas of infected rodents. Changes in sanitary conditions that would eliminate shelter or food for potential rodent vectors are possible long-term solutions. Killing all the organisms and all the fleas carried by these organisms would not be practical or desirable.

EARLY MEANS OF PREVENTION

In the past, many of the same types of remedies that were thought to be useful in treating the plague were sometimes used to prevent it. In keeping with the belief that the disease was spread through the air, many preventive measures involved odor. It was thought that if one carried flowers or wore a strong perfume, the odors would help keep away the disease. People believed carrying a lucky charm could ward off the disease, although there is no indication what that charm should consist of. Smoke from pipes was thought to repel the disease. After the year 1350, plague patients were placed in so-called pesthouses, where people with diseases were isolated from the general population. Ships coming from plague-infested areas were quarantined for 40 days until the disease could die out.

CURRENT MEANS OF PREVENTION

Almost every brochure, magazine, medical pamphlet, or Web site about the plague will suggest the same type of advice regarding prevention. To reduce the risk of contracting the plague, food sources and possible nest sites used by rodents should be eliminated. Every attempt should be made to rodent-proof homes, buildings, warehouses, or feed sheds. Chemicals that kill fleas and rodents are effective but can also cause health risks to humans and, therefore, should usually be applied by trained professionals. Trained professionals who can, if necessary, fumigate cargoes should inspect ships and docks. It is imperative that individuals avoid handling wild and domestic animals such as rats, cats, rabbits, and squirrels, especially in the western part of the United States. It is a good idea to avoid handling *any* sick or dead animal. Hunters should always wear gloves. Pets should receive weekly flea treatments with flea powder (especially in areas where plague is present).

People should stay away from areas that are known to harbor rats or seem likely to harbor rats. If people anticipate that they might be exposed to rodent fleas, they should apply a permethrin-containing repellent to clothing, shoes, and all camping gear. Permethrin is a synthetic broad-spectrum insecticide, similar to pyrethrin, a naturally occurring insecticide. Ineffective when applied to your skin, permethrin is very effective and durable on clothing and gear.

Insect repellants that contain N,N-diethyl-m-toluamide (DEET) should be applied to the skin and to clothing. However, because of toxicity, only formulations containing around 30% DEET should be used. DEET products should not be applied to infants under two months of age or to women who are pregnant or breastfeeding. DEET is designed for direct application to human skin to repel rather than kill insects. DEET was developed by the U.S. Army in 1946 and was registered for use by the public in 1957. Approximately 230 products containing DEET are currently registered with the EPA by about 70 different companies.

For those who have been exposed to animals infected with the plague bacterium or who must be present in an area where plague is present in the animal population, it is advisable to begin treatment with prophylactic antibiotics. Antibiotics such

BUBONIC PLAGUE HITS SAN FRANCISCO 1900–1909

On March 6, 1900, an autopsy on a dead Chinese man in San Francisco, California, revealed organisms that resembled those that cause plague. Despite public officials' immediate concerns over the potential health threat this discovery might pose, there were political issues that hampered them from taking immediate action. At the time, anti-Chinese sentiment was running strong. Many whites disliked the Chinese immigrants, who were blamed for taking jobs away from white American workers.

Upon finding plague in the dead man, San Francisco officials decided to quarantine Chinatown, the section of the city where most of the Chinese population lived. Both Chinese residents and members of the business community protested, although the businesses were worried more about the effects that the idea of plague in their city would have on business than about the rights of the Chinese. The city ended the quarantine, but instead carried out inspections of each house in Chinatown. Eventually, two more people were found to have died from plague.

At this point, the city made a formal announcement that there was an outbreak of plague in San Francisco. The governor of California refused to acknowledge the announcement, so, in order to take some action, the U.S. Surgeon General obtained presidential permission to enact laws to help stop the plague.

Still, the state's officials refused to admit there was a problem, and in the meantime, additional cases of plague turned up. Only in 1903, when a new governor came to office, was a concentrated effort made to help the board of health put an end to the epidemic. By February 29, 1904, when a woman from Concord, California, died of plague, the epidemic was over—at least temporarily. The area had counted 121 cases in the city of San Francisco and 5 outside, with a total of 122 deaths.

A few cases of plague were reported again in 1907, but this time, San Francisco, as well as other cities, were better prepared (Figure 6.1). Officials offered rewards for people who killed or captured potentially infected rats. This method, which worked well, was later used by other cities and states to help control outbreaks of plague.

Source: Available online at *http://www.pbs.org/wgbh/aso/databank/ entries/dm00bu.html.*

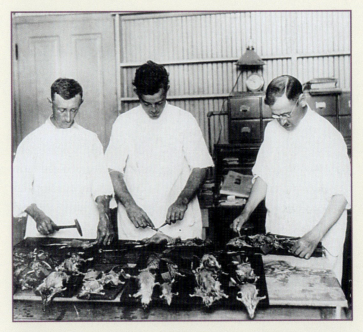

Figure 6.1 Although the outbreak of plague in San Francisco in 1900–1909 received the most publicity, it was not the only situation in which public health officials feared they were facing a dangerous plague epidemic. In 1914, the city of New Orleans, Louisiana, had a plague outbreak. These scientists are examining the bodies of dead rats to determine whether they were carriers of bubonic plague, in the hope of stopping the spread of the disease.

as doxycycline or tetracycline or any of the sulfonamides are recommended.

VACCINATION

Unfortunately, there is no **vaccine** against plague currently available in the United States (Figure 6.3). A licensed vaccine was available until the manufacturer discontinued its production in 1999 for financial reasons. This vaccine had been used against bubonic plague transmitted by fleabites but did not protect against pneumonic plague. Though data about the effectiveness of this vaccine are limited, the vaccination did seem to provide protection for military personnel during the Vietnam War. The vaccine caused antibody production against the F1 capsular antigen. New vaccine development is currently aimed at using live, **attenuated** strains of the bacterium (*Yersinia pestis*) or, more commonly, developing vaccines that target specific molecules on the cell surface of the plague organism.

However, in January 2003, the U.S. Defense Department granted Avant Immunotherapeutics Incorporated of Needham, Massachusetts, a contract worth $8 million to develop an oral vaccine against *Yersinia pestis* and *Bacillus anthracis*, the causative agent of anthrax. This vaccine is being developed to provide military personnel fast-acting protection against these two potential agents of biochemical warfare. Avant will not only design the vaccine but will also carry out all of the necessary laboratory investigations prior to human testing.

In the March 2003 issue of *Vaccine*, a veterinary products company named Heska published research about a vaccine to prevent the spread of plague in animals. The company had previously worked with the U.S. Geological Survey's National Wildlife Health Center on an experimental vaccine to prevent plague in prairie dogs. The new vaccine uses the same technique as the vaccine used to immunize mice against plague. The research is designed to develop a vaccine that would be

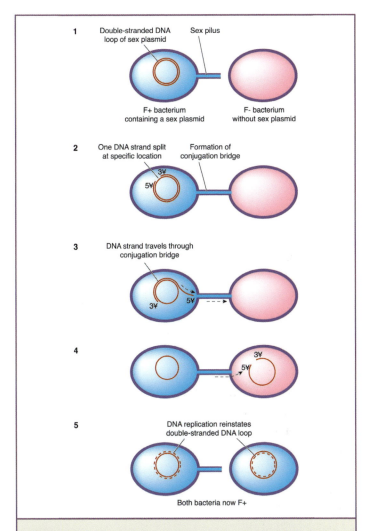

Figure 6.2 This diagram shows how a host cell that has already been infected by a bacterium spreads the disease it carries. First, it transfers plasmids horizontally to an uninfected cell (1) via the sex pilus, which serves as a bridge between the two cells. Then, the infected cell uses the "bridge" to send DNA that carries the infection to the other cell. Once inside the other cell, the DNA replicates, making the previously uninfected cell a precise copy of the cell that gave it the infection.

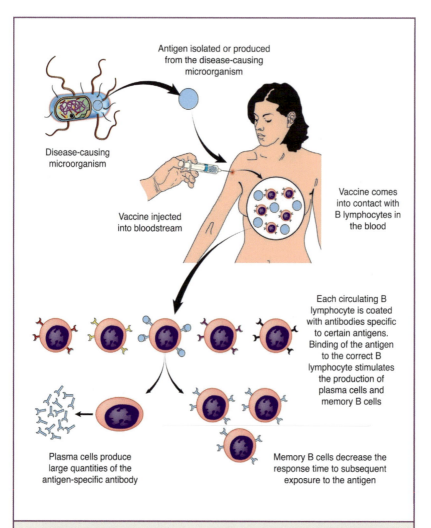

Antigen isolated or produced
from the disease-causing
microorganism

Disease-causing
microorganism

Vaccine injected
into bloodstream

Vaccine comes
into contact with
B lymphocytes in
the blood

Each circulating B
lymphocyte is coated
with antibodies specific
to certain antigens.
Binding of the antigen
to the correct B
lymphocyte stimulates
the production of
plasma cells and
memory B cells

Plasma cells produce
large quantities of the
antigen-specific antibody

Memory B cells decrease the
response time to subsequent
exposure to the antigen

Figure 6.3 Vaccination is one of the most useful ways to prevent infectious disease. In fact, it has helped doctors to virtually wipe out some diseases, such as polio and smallpox. This illustration shows how a vaccine is created and applied: First, the vaccine is made from a weakened or killed **antigen**. Then, it is injected into a person's bloodstream, where the immune system attacks and creates antibodies to the antigen. Thanks to the immune system's memory cells, the person is then protected against infection by the particular antigen in the future.

delivered orally to wild animal populations by embedding it in food left as bait in areas frequented by rodents.

VACCINES OUTSIDE THE UNITED STATES

Although it is not available in the United States, a vaccine against bubonic plague is manufactured and is available in some countries, including Australia. The plague vaccine can be given to both adults and children. For adults and children older than 12 years of age, two doses of the vaccine are needed and are given one to four weeks apart. Children under 12 years of age require three doses of the vaccine spaced one to four weeks apart. To achieve the possibility of full protection, all doses must be received. It takes the body several weeks to develop a sufficient supply of antibodies to assure protection. Even then, the vaccine cannot ensure 100% protection against the disease. People who live in areas where plague is active and widespread should receive a vaccine booster shot every six months. Other groups of individuals who should consider vaccination include people who work in the laboratory or in the field with the plague organism, including veterinary doctors and staff working with potentially infected animals.

7

The Problems of Antibiotic Resistance

Antibiotics are chemicals produced by living organisms, usually fungi or bacteria, that destroy or inhibit other microorganisms or their ability to reproduce. Since the mid-1950s, an increasing number of microbes have shown **antibiotic resistance**, and are no longer killed or inhibited by particular antibiotics. The initial relief that came from the ability to conquer disease through use of antibiotics such as penicillin and streptomycin has become muted as more microbes have found ways to neutralize or inactivate the antibiotics. The National Academy of Sciences has suggested that it may cost as much as $30 billion annually to treat antibiotic-resistant infections.

Microorganisms have lived in close proximity to each other in the soil and water for millions of years. Often, they compete for the same scarce resources. To succeed in such a competitive environment, microorganisms find biochemical means of destroying or inactivating chemicals produced by other organisms. This ongoing process in which one organism produces destructive chemicals and another finds ways to destroy the first organism is nature's way of maintaining a balance among the microbes in the soil and water.

The two main issues to address regarding antibiotic resistance are why and how it occurs.

WHY RESISTANCE OCCURS

Simply put, antibiotic resistance develops due to the abuse, misuse, and overuse of antibiotics. For example, antibiotics are ineffective against viruses, yet patients often press their doctors to prescribe antibiotics for viral maladies, including colds or influenza. If antibiotics are taken for a viral infection, they destroy some of the helpful bacteria in the intestines. Bacteria, both "good" and "bad," are in constant competition in the intestines. Destruction of the "good" bacteria provides opportunity for the unfettered growth of "bad" bacteria.

Another reason antibiotic resistance occurs is the failure of the patient to follow instructions. When antibiotics are prescribed, the patient is directed to take all of the antibiotics provided. Often, patients stop taking antibiotics as soon as they start to feel better, even though there are still bacteria in their bodies. By not completing a full course of antibiotics, only the least resistant of the offending bacteria are killed off, leaving the most resistant alive. These more resistant bacteria survive and reproduce, which means that the next time the person is infected, it will take a higher dosage or a different antibiotic to kill the same bacteria.

Microorganisms also can become resistant to antibiotics when antibiotics are used in low doses in livestock and agriculture. Antibiotics are often mixed with animal feed. The amounts are too small to be used for treating a disease, but they do destroy the least hardy bacteria. The most resistant bacteria survive. Part of the rationale for giving antibiotics to livestock is to keep the animals healthy and allow them to grow rapidly without competition from internal parasites in the form of intestinal bacteria. Antibiotic residues are also often found on fruits and vegetables that have been sprayed to reduce premature decomposition. If we are not careful about washing fruits and vegetables before we eat them, we may kill off some of our useful bacteria, allowing the more resistant and harmful organisms to survive. On June 3, 2002, *The New York Times* documented the discovery of the antibiotic chloramphenicol in shrimp imported from Asia. Agricultural use of this antibiotic is banned in the United States because it has been shown to cause problems such as childhood leukemia. So far, officials say that only a small percentage of the imported shrimp has been found to contain trace amounts of this antibiotic. However, its presence in food is a serious concern.

Finally, antibiotics may be available without a prescription in some countries. If a person taking an antibiotic is not aware of the limitations and potential problems that can occur when some bacteria survive antibiotic treatment, an environment may be created in which resistant organisms not only survive a course of antibiotics, but also grow more and more resistant over time.

HOW RESISTANCE DEVELOPS

Microorganisms have an amazing ability to adapt very rapidly to new and changing environmental conditions. They often have a reproductive rate that doubles their numbers in minutes. Both *Escherichia coli* and *Staphylococcus aureus* can double their numbers every 12 to 20 minutes under optimal conditions.

Bacteria have genetic material that is extremely flexible. It consists of a single chromosome and a number of small chunks of DNA called plasmids, which look like miniature chromosomes. Plasmids contain a limited number of genes that are often genetic codes for enzymes and other proteins that provide resistance to one or more antibiotics.

There are a number of ways that bacteria can develop resistance to antibiotics. One of these methods is through mutations of their genetic information or DNA. A **mutation** is a change in the genetic information of a cell or virus. A single mutation can spread through a population of bacteria in a matter of hours. If that mutation provides a way for bacteria to survive in the presence of a particular antibiotic, the genetic change will soon be found in millions of newly resistant bacteria. When bacteria die, other bacteria often scavenge the DNA of the dead microbe and incorporate it into their own genetic programs. Called **transformation**, this new information may contain genetic codes for inactivating or neutralizing various antibiotics.

Some bacteria can exchange copies of plasmids. A copy of a plasmid is passed through a protein tube called a pilus into another bacterium, during a process called conjugation, making it possible to exchange genetic information between live bacteria (Figure 7.1).

In a sense, this was the first information highway; it has been active for millions, perhaps billions, of years. Some of this new genetic information may provide the recipient bacterium with a competitive advantage in its environment.

Bacteria often are infected by specific viruses. As a virus infects one bacterium, it takes over the cell and forces the bacterium to produce and assemble new virus parts. As the new virus is constructed, it may incorporate some of the bacterial DNA into its own genetic program. When the new viruses infect other bacteria, they may leave some of the incorporated bacterial DNA in the newly infected bacterium. This process is called **transduction** and, like the others mentioned earlier, this method provides new genetic information to a bacterium that may allow it to become resistant to one or more antibiotics.

Bacteria have evolved a number of mechanisms at the molecular level that allow them to resist antibiotics.

- Often, an antibiotic must attach to a particular structure such as the cell wall or a protein receptor in the cell membrane. If the bacterium changes the target molecule in some way, the antibiotic will not be able to attach to the bacterium and will be ineffective.

- Some bacteria take the antibiotic into their cells and surround it with a membrane of proteins. This effectively prevents the antibiotic from interfering with a biochemical process or locking on to a receptor molecule.

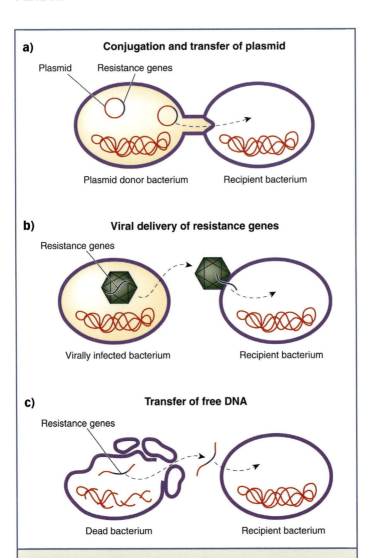

a) **Conjugation and transfer of plasmid**

Plasmid   Resistance genes

Plasmid donor bacterium   Recipient bacterium

b) **Viral delivery of resistance genes**

Resistance genes

Virally infected bacterium   Recipient bacterium

c) **Transfer of free DNA**

Resistance genes

Dead bacterium   Recipient bacterium

Figure 7.1 Bacteria can transfer its antibiotic resistance in three ways. In the process of conjugation (a), a bacterium injects its mutated genes into another bacterium through a special connection. A virus can also give its resistance genes to a new bacterium in a process known as transduction (b). Resistance genes can also be integrated into a new bacterium when another bacterium dies, in a process called transformation (c).

- Certain bacteria produce chemicals such as enzymes that inactivate or destroy the drug. One example is gonorrhea microbes that produce a chemical called penicillinase, which neutralizes penicillin. These microbes are designated penicillinase-producing *Neisseria gonorrhea* (PPNG).

- Other species of bacteria may contain structures, such as a capsule, which keep the antibiotic from penetrating into the cell.

- Some bacteria have molecular pumps called efflux systems that actively remove antibiotics or other unwanted chemicals from the cell.

CURRENT RESEARCH

A group of researchers at Old Dominion University in Norfolk, Virginia, has developed a way to study the efflux mechanisms of specific gram-negative bacteria. Efflux systems are designed to pump out of the bacterial cell substances such as antibiotics that the cell considers harmful. Dr. X. Nancy Xu and her colleagues from the department of chemistry and biochemistry combined two types of microscopy with a fluorescent dye called ethidium bromide. Their method allows for real-time study of individual live cells for an extended period.

The group found that individual cells vary greatly in the rate at which they pump out the antibiotics. Since the usual study method is to look at what happens with the majority of cells, being able to see individual cell differences will allow for earlier detection of the resistance. The short-term goal of the group is to understand the nature of multidrug resistance in the bacteria so that new therapies and drugs that target the pump mechanisms may be developed. "The purpose of this understanding of multidrug resistance is to be able to use a very low dose of drugs, for fewer side effects," said Dr. Xu. Xu suggested that the group also hopes to use this knowledge to construct and bioengineer an efflux pump that could possibly sense and deliver drugs.

The National Institute of Allergy and Infectious Diseases (NIAID) is a component of the National Institutes of Health (NIH). A major part of its job is to support research efforts to prevent, diagnose, and treat infectious and immune-mediated illnesses. NIAID supports research to study the molecular mechanisms responsible for drug resistance and to develop new chemical interventions for disease treatment and prevention. Since 1992, its research funding for antimicrobial resistance research has nearly doubled to nearly $14 million.

Research using gene-sequencing techniques can identify the critical molecules involved in microbial reproduction. These molecules may then serve as targets for new drugs. Research conducted so far in the area of drug resistance has led to:

- The discovery of methods that will make it possible to reverse resistance to antibiotics.

- An understanding of the genetic reasons why some parasites become resistant and the ability to recognize the organisms that are, in fact, resistant.

- New molecular level mechanisms and tools that make it easier to recognize those species that are resistant to specific drugs.

- New drugs being created to combat the drug-resistant strains of *Plasmodium*, the organism responsible for the disease malaria.

An editorial by David Dennis and James Hughes, both from the CDC, appeared in the September 4, 1997, issue of the *New England Journal of Medicine.* In the editorial, Dennis and Hughes addressed the problems associated with emerging infections, particularly with respect to growing antibiotic resistance in the plague bacillus and other bacteria carried by a

AN ANTIBIOTIC-RESISTANT PLAGUE ORGANISM

In 1995, a 16-year-old boy in Madagascar was diagnosed with bubonic plague. The particular strain isolated from the boy was identified as 17/95 biotype orientalis. This particular strain was resistant to eight different antibiotics, including ampicillin, chloramphenicol, kanamycin, streptomycin, spectinomycin, the sulfonamides, tetracycline, and minocycline. Resistance to most of these antibiotics was the result of the bacteria being able to produce chemicals that neutralized or inactivated the antibiotics.

Genetic analysis of the plasmid DNA found in the 17/95 strain showed that the plasmid contained fragments of another plasmid normally found in *Escherichia coli*, a normal intestinal bacillus. This brings up the question of how and where the *Y. pestis* bacteria acquired the *E. coli* plasmid. There are a number of places where both microbes would be found together, including inside and outside the mammalian host. Of greater concern is the fact that plasmids are transferable between species, increasing the likelihood that more multidrug-resistant *Y. pestis* will appear again.

In October 2002, the question of how and where *Yersinia* acquired the *E. coli* plasmid appeared to be answered. A group of researchers showed that *Yersinia* acquires antibiotic-resistant plasmids from *E. coli* by horizontal transfer within the midgut of the flea. It is clear from the article that close physical contact between the *E. coli* and the *Y. pestis* plasmids leads to high-frequency conjugative genetic exchange. The article suggests that this may have been the source of the antibiotic-resistant strain isolated from the boy in Madagascar.

variety of vectors such as fleas, ticks, flies, and mosquitoes. They suggest that the first line of defense against these emerging diseases would be a system of domestic and global **surveillance** and response. Dennis and Hughes further indicated that there are four basic requirements for such a system. The first would be the ability to detect clusters of new and unusual diseases and syndromes. Second would be the capability to identify and characterize the infectious agents in a laboratory setting. Third is the ability to analyze and distribute information quickly and globally. Fourth would be the development of feedback systems that would cause both investigative and control responses. Hughes and Dennis suggest that each of these four components is "critical in confronting the emergence of plague and the potential for the emergence of drug-resistant disease."

The editorial was written in response to another article also appearing in the same issue. The article, entitled "Multidrug Resistance in *Yersinia pestis* Mediated by a Transferable Plasmid," was written by Marc Garlimand and six of his colleagues. The article points out that plague is now considered a reemerging disease and, since 1994, has appeared in epidemic numbers in at least three countries. The plague organism is normally susceptible to a number of antibiotics including streptomycin, chloramphenicol, tetracycline, and the sulfonamides.

8

Concerns for the Future

There are two major interrelated concerns that seem to override all others when it comes to the plague: (1) the concern that new, antibiotic-resistant strains of the organism will become common; and (2) the concern that the plague organism might be used as a weapon of bioterrorism.

EVOLUTION OF RESISTANT STRAINS

As discussed in Chapter 7, increasing antibiotic resistance is a major problem in dealing with disease organisms such as *Yersinia pestis*. One of the major reasons that *Y. pestis* survives in the environment of the flea's midgut is because it has an enzyme called phospholipase D (PLD). This enzyme, formerly called *Yersinia* murine toxin, gives the microbe resistance to a product in the blood plasma of the flea that would otherwise destroy the bacterium. It is still not known exactly what molecular mechanisms provide this protection. *Yersinia pestis* acquired the gene for production of PLD from either an unrelated bacterium or a simple nucleated organism such as a protozoan. Once *Y. pestis* had acquired this gene, it had a new means of transmission. The bacteria transformed from an organism that caused mild stomach illness through contaminated food and water to a flea-borne carrier of a life-threatening disease. The evolution of *Y. pestis* also shows how microbes are constantly reemerging in new forms and in new ways as agents of disease.

HISTORY OF PLAGUE AS A WEAPON

It has been suggested that plague served as the original biological weapon in wartime. History records that the Tatars were attempting to capture the Italian-controlled city of Kaffa on the shore of the Black Sea in 1347.

Plague broke out in the Tatar camp. The defenders of Kaffa resisted until the Tatars began to hurl the bodies of their own dead over the walls and into the city. The Tatars had been dying

GLOBAL OUTBREAK ALERT AND RESPONSE NETWORK

In April 2000, the World Health Organization (WHO) set up a meeting between representatives of technical institutions, various organizations, and networks involved in surveillance and response to global epidemics. The participants recognized the need to provide a global network to identify and deal with the threats posed by epidemic-prone and emerging diseases. This newly formed network developed a set of *Guiding Principles for International Outbreak Alert and Response*. In addition, they have developed laboratory rules and regulations that provide standardization in various areas such as research, communications, security, and clinical management.

The Global Outbreak Alert and Response Network uses technical and other resources from the scientific groups within WHO. In addition, it has partnered with United Nations organizations such as UNICEF, the Red Cross, and international humanitarian organizations worldwide. This network works towards providing security to global health by:

- Combating the international spread of outbreaks.

- Ensuring that appropriate technical assistance reaches affected states rapidly.

- Contributing to long-term epidemic preparedness and capacity building.

Since its inception, the network has been involved in projects in at least 19 different countries from Afghanistan to Uganda, dealing with diseases including yellow fever, influenza, Ebola fever, and Rift Valley fever.

by the thousands of the plague, and now, so did the defenders of the city. Those who eventually escaped the city took to their ships and headed for ports in the Mediterranean, carrying the plague with them. The city of Kaffa became uninhabitable, and the Black Death quickly spread throughout Europe.

During World War II, the Japanese were known to have dropped fleas infected with plague organisms over populated areas of China. A number of outbreaks of plague resulted. After World War II, both the United States and the Soviet Union used their biological weapons programs to find new techniques and delivery methods for a variety of microbial agents, including plague. Both countries were successful in finding ways to aerosolize *Yersinia pestis*, which increased its usefulness as a potential biological weapon.

Obviously, this ability to spread the organism in an aerosol form has led to concern that terrorist groups or nations might acquire and use it. Scientists who defected from the former Soviet Union suggested that an antibiotic-resistant strain of *Yersinia pestis* had been developed.

In 2001, the complete genome of the plague microbe was sequenced. Julian Parkhill, leader of the sequencing team, suggested that the sequence would be critical in helping to design antibiotics and vaccines that may be used against this disease organism. Another member of the group, Rick Titball, is leading a team that has produced a vaccine that is currently in **clinical trials**. Titball believes that "The information available [about the genome] is of much greater advantage to people defending against biological warfare than to those intending to use it."

PLAGUE AS A BIOTERRORIST AGENT

The CDC has placed plague in Category A, which is the highest priority category for an agent that could be used for bioterrorist activity. It meets the criteria set up by the CDC, which are that:

- It is easily disseminated or transmitted from person to person,

- It results in high mortality rate and has the potential for major public health impact,

- It might cause panic or social disruption,

- It requires special action for public health preparedness.

The Working Group on Civilian Biodefense prepared a consensus statement that concluded:

Given the availability of *Y. pestis* around the world, capacity for its mass production and aerosol dissemination, difficulty in preventing such activities, high fatality rate of pneumonic plague, and potential for secondary spread of cases during an epidemic, the potential use of plague as a biological weapon is of great concern.

In 1970, the WHO issued a report suggesting that up to 36,000 deaths and more than 150,000 incapacitating illnesses would result from the airborne release of 50 kilograms (approximately 110 pounds) of dried powder containing *Yersinia pestis* in a country such as the United States. These numbers represent only direct impacts and do not take into account the number of secondary infections and deaths that would result from subsequent person-to-person contact.

NIAID RESEARCH

Because bioterrorism continues to be a real concern for the United States, NIAID and other agencies have accelerated microbial research and development of diagnostic, preventive, and treatment methods. Microbial **genomics**, the study of the totality of genetic information found in an organism, has become an important part of this overall approach. The complete collection of an organism's genetic information is known as its **genome**. Understanding an organism's genetic program may aid in understanding how an organism carries out its biochemical and physical processing and operates as a complex biological system.

This genetic information can be used "to develop gene-based diagnostic and sampling tests to quickly detect dangerous germs and assess their susceptibility to different types of treatment. Genomes also provide molecular fingerprints of different strains of a given microbe, thereby enabling investigators to better track future outbreaks to their source." Current long-term research of NIAID includes:

- Identifying genes in the *Y. pestis* bacterium that infect the digestive tract of fleas and researching how the bacterium is transferred to humans.

- Studying the disease-causing proteins and genes of *Y. pestis* that allow the bacterium to grow in humans and how they function in human lungs.

NIAID is also working with the Department of Defense, the CDC, and the Department of Energy to:

- Develop a vaccine that protects against inhalationally acquired pneumonic plague (Figure 8.1).

- Develop promising antibiotics and intervention strategies to prevent and treat plague infection.

In 2002, NIAID released its "Biodefense Research Agenda for CDC Category A Agents." The bubonic plague organism was high on the list of the greatest bioterror threats.

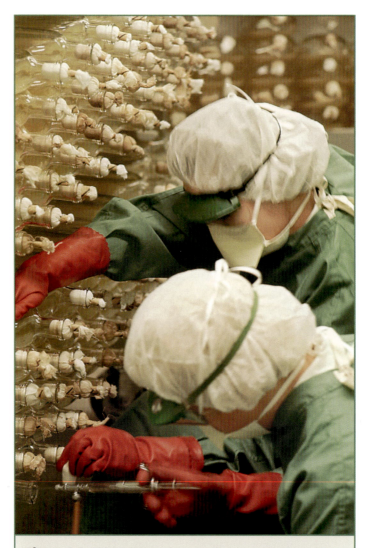

Figure 8.1 Although there is currently no vaccine in use to prevent bubonic plague in the United States, working vaccines have been created in the past, which lends hope that they could be used in the future if ever a pressing need arose. In fact, research is always being done (as these scientists demonstrate) to find a useful, cost-effective vaccine for plague. In the meantime, most cases of plague are treated successfully with antibiotics.

A FINAL CAUTION

Bubonic plague, though not a problem in most of the country, can become a nightmare for those who are infected by it. In the opening chapter, a couple from New Mexico, John Tull and his wife, Lucinda Marker, became sick with bubonic plague while visiting New York City. What started out as a vacation turned into a near-death experience. Although Lucinda recovered quickly, John nearly died and had to spend 227 days in the hospital. For three months of that time, he was in a coma. His feet became gangrenous and both of his legs were amputated below the knee. Once he was released from the New York City hospital, he spent time in the Rehabilitation Center of New Mexico. John is making a remarkable recovery but he must be monitored continuously. He is still receiving therapy three times a week. His is just one more life altered by the bubonic plague.

9

Hopes for the Future

Techniques originally used to help analyze the human genome may soon be used as tools to decipher the DNA of *Y. pestis*, investigate how antibiotic resistance develops, and make earlier detection possible. Researchers are also looking at ways to investigate a number of host-pathogen interactions, including how pathogens use host cell membrane proteins to enter host cells.

DETECTING BACTERIAL DNA SEQUENCES

Antibiotic resistance in bacteria is an inherited characteristic, but attempting to analyze all of the DNA of all of the organisms present in an infection is not practical. A new method is under development at the University of Rochester Medical Center in Rochester, New York, that detects the presence of specific DNA sequences. Certain portions of DNA molecules take particular shapes based on their ability to find a complementary information sequence at the end of the DNA molecule. Once the DNA sequence that represents antibiotic resistance is found in one bacterial species, that sequence can be used as a model to find the same sequence in other bacteria. A fluorescent molecule is attached to one end of the DNA strand and can be used as a molecular beacon when bacteria suspected of being antibiotic-resistant are checked on a slide. The hope is that a single microarray or DNA chip would be able to test different species as well as different strains within a species to determine if they are resistant to a specific antibiotic.

DISCOVERING HOW TO DISABLE BACTERIAL WEAPONS

In May 1999, researchers announced that they had found a way to prevent a number of bacteria from causing disease. It is hoped that the findings, published in the journal *Science*, can be used to develop a new generation of vaccines and antibiotics. The researchers reported that they had identified a "master switch" that controls the production of many chemicals that bacteria use to cause infection. When they knock out the switch, the bacteria are no longer capable of causing disease. It seems that the master switch for pathogenic bacteria, such as *Vibrio cholerae* (cholera), *Yersinia* (plague), *Salmonella* (typhoid fever), and *Shigella* (dysentery), is the same. Treatment of these

MICROARRAYS

Microarrays, also called DNA chips, gene chips, DNA micro-arrays, or gene expression microarrays, represent a blending of computer technology and DNA. Researchers cover a small glass chip with hundreds to thousands of fragments of DNA. Each of these fragments represents a different gene within the cell being studied. By adding a fluorescent molecule to the fragments, they can be made to light up when they come into contact with a complementary gene. This tells scientists about the activity level of the genes in question. Microarrays make it possible for researchers to determine which genes are being activated and under what conditions. These microarrays are being used to try to understand the genetics involved with how microorganisms respond to drugs, how they respond to different environmental conditions, and how they are able to infect different kind of host cells. This new technology gives us the opportunity to test many genes simultaneously, thus speeding up the process of detecting change within the cell.

Source: U.S. Department of Health and Human Services, National Institutes of Health, National Institute of Allergy and Infectious Diseases, Division of Microbiology and Infectious Diseases. "Deciphering Pathogens: Blueprints for New Medical Tools." NIH Publication No. 02-4987 (September 2002). Available online at *http://cmgm.stanford.edu/biochem/gfx/images/brown_arrayimage.jpg*.

bacterial infections, as well as others, may be affected by this discovery. It is also hoped that this discovery can be used in the fight against newly emerging, drug-resistant pathogens.

Michael Mahan and his colleagues used a mutated strain of *Salmonella* with the master switch always on. This allowed researchers to discover all the tricks the organisms use for getting past the stomach and intestines and into organs and tissues. "This [knowledge of how to stop organisms from invading] has two important consequences," Mahan states. "The bacteria are completely disabled in their ability to cause disease and these crippled bacteria work as a vaccine since they stimulate immune defenses to defend against subsequent infections."

DECIPHERING THE DNA OF *YERSINIA PESTIS*

Determining the sequence of the bubonic plague organism will hopefully lead to the design and development of new antibiotics and vaccines. In this case, we will also learn a great deal about how infectious bacteria have evolved over time. According to Brendan Wren, a member of the sequencing team, the plague organism descended from an intestinal organism, *Yersinia pseudotuberculosis*. "Two thousand years ago it gave you a mild tummy ache," says Wren. One reason for the rapid evolution of *Y. pestis* may be its ability to shuffle segments of its chromosome, an activity common among pathogens. *Yersinia pestis* also carries genes for insecticidal toxins that are now deactivated but may have aided its move into the fleas. The *Y. pestis* organism contains about 150 pseudogenes—repeating, gene-like sequences of DNA that are no longer active in the organism. These sequences may eventually be lost from the organism completely.

HOW BACTERIAL CELLS COMMUNICATE

Biologists have long speculated that bacteria are able to communicate with each other and their environment by releasing and then detecting various types of chemicals. This activity is a form of molecular census-taking and is usually called quorum sensing. Evidence exists that indicates more than 70 different types of organisms, including *Yersinia pestis*, are engaged in this activity. According to researcher Rong-guang Zhang, "We believe the quorum-sensing process signals bacteria to create biofilms—mats of bacterial cells over a solid surface."

The researchers used the Structural Biology Laboratory at Argonne National Laboratories to determine the molecular structure of a protein called *TraR*. This key protein seems to act as a relay that senses chemicals called pheromones. Once the bacterial cell senses these molecules, it activates specific genes that allow it to create biofilms. Knowing the structure of this protein allows scientists to pursue two different avenues of research. They may be able to find or create drugs that would block the chemical signals and thus prevent formation of biofilms. Conversely, they could stimulate the production of biofilms for useful projects such as water filtration.

NEW ANTIBACTERIAL DRUGS

Researchers at the Wistar Institute in Philadelphia have identified and isolated a group of insect peptides (short proteins) that attack specific molecules in bacteria. Insects lack an immune system and have devised strategies to eliminate bacteria and other germs. The insect host may use peptides to create holes in bacterial membranes, or the peptides may bind to target sites within the bacterial cells causing death in some poorly understood way. Working with a European sap-sucking insect, *Pyrrhocoris apterus,* scientists identified the antimicrobial peptide called pyrrhocoricin. The target of this molecule is another protein called *DnaK* whose job is to identify and correct the shape of proteins that have folded up incorrectly. *DnaK* is a "heat-shock protein" and, when it is bound by the pyrrhocoricin, *DnaK* is unable to complete its work of repairing misshapen proteins. This usually leads to the death of the bacterium. The insect peptide does not bind to mouse or human equivalents of *DnaK* and thus is not toxic to humans.

NANOPARTICLES CAN BE USED TO KILL BACTERIA

Researchers at Kansas State University have developed nanoparticles made of magnesium oxide to kill various bacteria, including bioterrorism agents such as anthrax and *E. coli*, in about five minutes. Kenneth J. Klabunde and his team have shown that these particles have an electrical charge opposite to that of the electrical charge on bacteria. The opposite charges attract the particles to the bacteria. The sharp edges of the particles penetrate even endospores of anthrax bacteria. Because the particles are alkaline rather than acidic, they can penetrate bacterial cell walls. Nanoparticles are solid rather than gaseous or liquid, which would allow them to be placed in air filtration units or sprayed like a powder.

NEW DIAGNOSTIC TESTS

The ability to detect the plague organism rapidly would greatly reduce the number of deaths and the likelihood of transmission among people. Scientists from the Pasteur Institute in France and the Ministry of Health in Madagascar developed a simple test, called a dipstick test, that provides reliable results within 15 minutes. The dipstick test recognizes a unique substance called F1 antigen, which is found in the blood and infected fluid of buboes. By rapid detection of pneumonic plague, more infected patients will be able to get rapid treatment. According to David Dennis and May C. Chu, the test "is expected to fill an important need in bioterrorism preparedness and response."

NEW VACCINES

The United States Department of Health and Human Services established eight Centers of Excellence for Biodefense and Emerging Infectious Diseases Research. Scientists from the Fred Hutchinson Cancer Research Center in Seattle, Washington, will be involved in developing vaccines for diseases that pose significant threats to public health. Dr. Nina Salama will lead the center's research attempting to identify potential vaccine targets for *Yersinia pestis*. Salama will work with Dr. Jeff Delrow in developing tools for analyzing bacterial genomes. Salama is using techniques and strategies she developed to study the ulcer-causing bacterium *Helicobacter pylori*. She identifies bacterial genes used by the bacteria to cause disease and that become highly activated during the course of the disease. These genes cause production of specific proteins that can be purified and then tested to see if they initiate an immune response when injected into a test animal. "The idea is to find proteins that are made in abundance by the bacteria when it infects an animal—which are the most likely proteins to provoke an immune response—but that also are absolutely necessary for the bacteria to cause illness," said Salama. The researchers will use the new gene-scanning tool called a DNA microarray.

Salama and Delrow had already constructed microarrays for their work with *Helicobacter pylori*, the bacterium responsible for most stomach ulcers. These arrays will identify highly reactive genes and compare their activity to arrays with individual gene mutations within different strains of *Yersinia*. In this way, they hope to find whichever strains are no longer capable of infection.

NEW VACCINE TRIALS

Currently in clinical trials is a new type of vaccine for the plague. At this point, vaccines do not provide 100% protection against the inhaled forms of the plague. Nose drops and nasal sprays of biodegradable microspheres containing antigenic subunits F1 and V are being tested on mice. This approach seems to protect the animals from inhaled and injected forms of the plague organism. Testing in larger animal models and humans will follow. This type of a vaccine has the advantage of being administered easily and to large numbers of people quickly. Another vaccine possibility involves the use of monoclonal antibodies against the V and F1 antigens of *Yersinia pestis*. Whether given alone or in combination, mice were protected against bubonic and pneumonic plague. The antibodies worked well whether given prior to infection or within 48 hours after infection.

NEW REGIONAL CENTERS
FOR BIODEFENSE RESEARCH

In September 2003, Tommy G. Thompson, secretary of Health and Human Services (HHS) announced that $350 million in grants was being released to establish eight Regional Centers of Excellence for Biodefense and Emerging Infectious Diseases Research (RCE). These centers will be part of the nation's plan for research in biodefense. "We have moved with unprecedented speed and determination to prepare for a bioterror attack or any other public health crisis since the terrorist attacks of 2001," Thompson said. "These new grants add to this effort and will not only better prepare us for a bioterrorism attack, but will also enhance our ability to deal with any public health crisis, such as SARS and West Nile virus."

The NIAID is providing the grants and will administer the RCE program. "Since the terrorist attacks on American soil in 2001, NIAID has moved rapidly to bolster basic biomedical research and the development of countermeasures to defend the United States against deliberately released agents of bioterrorism as well as naturally occurring infectious diseases," said Anthony S. Fauci, director of NIAID. "The new RCE program provides a coordinated and comprehensive mechanism to support the interdisciplinary research that will lead to new and improved therapies, vaccines, diagnostics and other tools to protect the citizens of our country and the world against the threat of bioterrorism and other emerging and re-emerging diseases."

All of the Regional Centers for Excellence will:

- Train researchers and other personnel for biodefense research activities.

- Create and maintain supporting resources, including scientific equipment and trained support personnel, for use by the RCEs and other researchers in the region.

- Emphasize research focused on development and testing of vaccine, therapeutic, and diagnostic concepts.

- Make available core facilities to approved investigators from academia, government, biotechnology companies, and the pharmaceutical industry.

- Provide facilities and scientific support to first responders in the event of a national biodefense emergency.

- Support investigator-directed research.

Each center comprises a lead institution and affiliated institutions located primarily in the same geographical region. The eight institutions receiving an RCE grant are: Duke University, Harvard Medical School, New York State Department of Health, University of Chicago, University of Maryland (Baltimore), University of Texas Medical Branch (Galveston), University of Washington, and Washington University in St. Louis. Research to be conducted in the RCE program includes:

- Developing new approaches to blocking the action of anthrax, botulinum, and cholera toxins.

- Developing new vaccines against anthrax, plague, tularemia, smallpox, and Ebola.

- Developing new antibiotics and other therapeutic strategies.

- Studying bacterial and viral disease processes.

- Designing new advanced diagnostic approaches for biodefense and for emerging diseases.

- Conducting immunological studies of diseases caused by potential agents of bioterrorism.

- Developing computational and genomic approaches to combating disease agents.

- Creating new immunization strategies and delivery systems.

In addition to the RCE, the NIAID will also fund construction of two National Biocontainment Laboratories (NBLs) and nine Regional Biocontainment Laboratories (RBLs). "These awards to build high-level biosafety facilities are a major step towards being able to provide Americans with effective therapies, vaccines and diagnostics for diseases caused by agents of bioterror as well as for naturally occurring emerging infections such as SARS and West Nile virus," said HHS Secretary Thompson.

The terrorist attacks of September 11, 2001, placed a new emphasis on improving and increasing our national health-care facilities. Plague is just one of the deadly diseases that has come to the attention of the public in the wake of 9/11. Scientists hope greater awarensss and additional research will help stop the plague once and for all.

Anaerobic—Not requiring oxygen.

Antibiotic—A chemical produced either by a microorganism such as a bacterium or a fungus such as a mold used to treat bacterial infections. Antibiotics are not useful in fighting viruses. Some antibiotics are currently produced synthetically either completely or in part (e.g., semi-synthetic penicillins such as ampicillin).

Antibiotic resistance—Also called drug resistance; the condition when organisms such as bacteria are no longer killed or inhibited by an antibiotic; the opposite of antibiotic sensitivity.

Antibody—An immune protein or immunoglobulin. These proteins are produced by white blood cells called lymphocytes. When stimulated by a foreign protein, chemical, or cell part, lymphocytes are converted into protein- (antibody-) producing factories.

Antigen—A molecule, group of molecules, or part of a cell that is recognized by the host immune cells as being *nonself* or foreign. Antigens stimulate production of antibodies (*anti*body *gen*erating).

Antiphagocytic—Unable to perform phagocytosis, or the prevention of phagocytosis.

Attenuated—Weakened.

Bacillus—When the term is used with a capital "B," it refers to a specific genus of bacteria that have a rod-like shape; when used with a lowercase "b," the term refers to the a rod-like shape (a rod is longer than it is wide).

Bipolar staining—Staining technique in which dye molecules concentrate at the ends or poles of the cells, giving them the appearance of a safety pin characteristic of *Yersinia* and *Franciscella* species.

Bubo—A swelling of the lymph nodes. Adjective form is *bubonic*.

Cholecystitis—Inflammation of the gallbladder that may be the result of infection in the gallbladder; gallstones may be present.

Clinical trials—Rigorous scientific evaluation of a procedure, device, or drug(s) used for prevention, diagnosis, or treatment of a disease. Usually three phases (Phases I, II, III) are required for approval by the Food and Drug Administration (FDA):

Phase I: Evaluation of clinical pharmacology, involves volunteers; testing for safety.

Glossary

Phase II: Performed in a small group of patients; testing for dosage and overall desired clinical effect.

Phase III: Large, comparative study using patients to establish a clear clinical benefit; control groups using placebos or comparisons to established or current procedures.

Coccus—Refers to shape of a bacterial cell that resembles a sphere or circle (plural is *cocci*). Staphylococcus (a cluster of cocci) and streptococcus (a chain of cocci) are common arrangements of specific groups of cocci well known for causing diseases.

Cytoskeleton—An internal protein framework inside eukaryotic cells.

Endemic—Refers to frequency of disease cases in a well-defined geographic region; frequency is low but cases are constantly present.

Endotoxin—A metabolic product released from the cell walls of gram-negative bacteria when they die. Composed of lipids, polysaccharides, and peptides, endotoxins are often toxic to the cells and may cause an inflammatory reaction.

Enzootic reservoirs—Populations of organisms that maintain a pathogenic organism, such as *Yersinia pestis*, within their population in low levels, resulting in low mortality.

Enzyme—A protein that serves as an organic catalyst, speeding up the rate of a biochemical reaction, but not consumed or used up in that reaction. All biochemical reactions within living systems are controlled or regulated by enzymes.

Epidemic—A dramatic increase in the number of individuals showing the symptoms of a disease within a specified area and during a specified time period. In the United States, statistics to determine a true epidemic are collected and maintained by the Centers for Disease Control and Prevention (CDC).

Epizootic reservoir—Population of organisms that are highly susceptible to a pathogen such as *Yersinia pestis*, with resulting high mortality.

Eukaryote, Eukaryotic—A type of cellular organization in which an organism contains a nucleus and one or more cells with a nucleus and other well-developed compartments known as organelles. These organelles consist of membranes or are bounded by membranes.

Facultative anaerobe—An organism that can grow and reproduce in the presence or absence of oxygen.

Flagellin—A protein that is used to construct the flagella of various bacteria.

Flagellum—A whip-like tail structure that helps a bacterium to move. Plural is *flagella*.

Free radical oxygen—Reactive by-products of metabolism; free radicals have only single electrons in their outer energy level and remove electrons from other molecules to complete their outer energy level; this electron stealing sets off a chain of biochemical events in the cells, creating instability that could destroy the cell.

GAP proteins—Proteins that activate an enzyme (GTPase) that breaks down an energy storage molecule known as GTP (guanine triphosphate), thus releasing energy to be used in various cellular activities.

Gastroenteritis—Inflammation of the stomach and the intestines; may result in nausea and vomiting and/or diarrhea.

Genetic or **gene mutation**—Change in the genetic information of a cell or virus (either DNA or RNA in some viruses); changes in genetic information usually lead to new proteins, altered proteins or loss of proteins.

Genome—The sum total of all the genetic information in a cell or virus.

Genomics—The study of the totality of genetic information found in an organism.

Glycoprotein—A molecule made of simple sugars such as glucose (glyco-) and a protein; commonly found on the outside of cell membranes and involved in cellular recognition and rejection.

Gram-negative—Refers to the designation given to bacteria that have been stained by the a Gram stain method. Gram-negative bacteria lose the color of the first or primary stain (crystal violet) and take the color of the second or counterstain (safranin—a red color). Thus, gram-negative cells are red to pink in color. The organisms responsible for typhoid fever, cholera, and bubonic plague are gram-negative.

Gram-positive—Refers to the designation given to bacteria that have been stained by the a Gram stain method. Gram-positive bacteria retain the color of the crystal violet stain due to the composition of the cell wall and thus are colored purple to violet.

Glossary

Inflammation—A series of responses consisting of redness, increased heat in the area, swelling, and pain; this is followed by repair of the inflamed area and is part of the nonspecific defenses of the body.

Invasin—A protein found on the outer membrane of certain bacteria, such as *Yersinia* species, which allows the bacteria to attach to the cell membrane of human cells.

Kinase—An enzyme involved in the transfer of phosphate groups on molecules.

Lipopolysaccharide (LPS)—A molecule composed of fatty acids and sugars, it makes up a portion of the cell wall of gram-negative bacteria such as *Yersinia*.

Lymphatic system—Includes the lymph nodes, spleen, tonsils, adenoids, and the thymus as well as scattered patches of tissue in various area of the body, such as the intestinal mesentery. The lymphatic tissue system is part of the body's immune system, producing cells that help protect the body from bacteria and other microbes.

Lymph nodes—Bean-shaped organs of the lymphatic system that contain various types of white blood cells and become swollen when infected.

Lymphocytes—One of the five types of white blood cells produced by humans; divided into B and T lymphocytes, both of which are essential to proper immune function.

Macrophage—A modified version of the monocyte, one of the five types of white blood cells in humans. A large cell that seeks out and engulfs foreign particles and cells through phagocytosis; literally, a "large eater."

Mutation—A change in the genetic information of a cell or virus (either DNA or RNA in some viruses). Changes in genetic information usually lead to new proteins, altered proteins, or loss of proteins.

Nonencapsulated—Lacking a capsule or envelope.

Organelles—"Miniature organs;" compartments within eukaryotic cells that are limited or bounded by membranes; they represent the sites of various metabolic actions and functions.

Pandemic—A worldwide epidemic or widespread disease in humans; it results when person-to-person contact occurs between individuals who have the virus but no current immune protection against it (these types of individuals are sometimes called "immunologically naïve").

Plasma—The liquid portion of the blood.

Plasmid—A small circle of DNA outside of the bacterial chromosome that is capable of self-replication. These miniature chromosomes carry a limited set of genes that can be copied and sent by means of protein tube from one bacterium to another, increasing the genetic variability of the recipient bacterium.

Pneumonic—Refers to the lungs; a form of plague that invades the lung tissue and is highly contagious.

Preclinical—Studies of drugs or vaccines that are carried out in tissue or cell cultures or animals; this phase occurs before clinical trials involving humans.

Prokaryote, Prokaryotic—A type of cellular organization in which cells lack membrane-enclosed organelles such as a nucleus; bacteria and archaea are prokaryotic cells.

Protease—An enzyme that can break down proteins.

Septicemic, septicemia—Referring to large numbers of bacteria in the bacterial infection of the bloodstream; sometimes known as blood poisoning.

Serology—The study of the serum.

Serum—The portion of the blood remaining after the blood cells, platelets, and proteins (the formed elements) have been removed.

Spirillum—A bacterium that is shaped like a spiral or curved like the letter "c."

Surveillance—A continuous and organized collection and analysis of data regarding all aspects of a disease. This information is sent to national and regional public health professionals, who use it to provide an up-to-date prevention and control program.

Sylvatic plague—Plague caused by organisms such as prairie dogs and squirrels, found in natural areas such as woodlands, grasslands, or forests, that carry the fleas that carry the plague organisms.

Transduction—A means by which bacteria acquire fragments of DNA and viruses transport DNA fragments from a donor cell to a recipient cell.

Glossary

Transformation—Alteration of the normal genetic information of a cell such as a bacterium by the inclusion of additional DNA from an outside source.

Urban plague—Plague caused by organisms such as rats, found in cities, that carry the fleas that carry the plague organisms.

Vaccine—A substance, organism, viral particle, or group of molecules that, when injected or put into the body by other means, will cause the immune system to mount an immune response to that specific agent.

Vectors—Organisms such as flies, fleas, and ticks that carry pathogenic organisms and transmit them to other organisms.

Bahmanyar, M., and D.C. Cavanaugh. *Plague Manual.* Geneva: World Health Organization, 1976.

Centers for Disease Control and Prevention. "Prevention of plague." Recommendations of the Advisory Committee on Immunization Practices (ACIP). *MMWR* 45 (RR-14) (1996): 1–15.

Craven, R.B., and D.T. Dennis. "Plague." *Maxcy-Rosenau-Last Public health and preventive medicine,* 14th ed., ed. R. B. Wallace. Stamford, CT: Appleton & Lange, 1998, pp. 309–313.

Gage, K.L. "Plague." *Topley and Wilson's microbiology and microbiological infections,* vol. 3, eds. L.A. Colliers, A. Balows, M. Sussman, and W.J. Hausles. London: Edward Arnold Press, 1998, pp. 885–903.

WEBSITES

Journal of the American Medical Association. "Plague as a Biological Weapon." **http://jama.ama-assn.org/cgi/content/full/283/17/2281.**

PBS Online. "People and Discoveries: A Science Odyssey." **http://www.pbs.org/wgbh/aso/databank/entries/dm00bu.html.**

Plague Prevention: Fact Sheet: Bubonic Plague. **http://www.responsiblewildlifemanagement.org/plague_prevention.htm.**

Sustainable Life. "Garlic." **http://www.sustlife.com/br4up/ASustlife/herbalremedies/garlic.htm.**

University of Maryland Medicine. "Bubonic Plague." **http://www.umm.edu/outdoor/bubonic_plague.htm.**

Further Reading

Centers for Disease Control and Prevention. "Basic Laboratory Protocols for the Presumptive Identification of *Yersinia pestis*." 4/18/2001.

Cornelis, Guy R. "Molecular and cell biology aspects of plague." *Proceedings of the National Academy of Sciences, USA* 97 (16) (2000): 8778–8783.

Garrett, Laurie. *Betrayal of Trust: The Collapse of Global Public Health.* New York: Hyperion Books, 2000.

———. *The Coming Plague: Newly Emerging Diseases in a World Out of Balance.* New York: Penguin Books, 1994.

Gottfried, R.S. *The Black Death: Natural and Human Disaster in Medieval Europe.* New York: The Free Press, 1983.

Gregory, Alicia P. "Countering Bioterror: The New Threat of the Plague." Available online at *http://www.rgs.uky.edu/ca/odyssey/fall02/plague.html.*

Inglesby, T. V., et al. "Plague as a biological weapon: Medical and public health management. Working Group on Civilian Biodefense." *Journal of the American Medical Association* 283 (17) (2000): 2281–1190.

"Prevention of Plague: Recommendations of the Advisory Committee on Immunization Practices (ACIP)." *Morbidity and Mortality Weekly Report* (CDC), vol. 45, December 13, 1996.

Centers for Disease Control and Prevention
www.cdc.gov

National Institute of Allergy and Infectious Diseases
www.niaid.nih.gov

National Institutes of Health
www.nih.gov

Website for John Tull
www.johnandlucinda.com/

World Health Organization
www.who.int

Index

Picture Credits

10: *Morbidity and Mortality Weekly Report*
    (MMWR), Vol. 52, No. 31, Courtesy CDC
15: Public Health Image Library (PHIL),
    Courtesy CDC
21: PHIL, Courtesy CDC
25: Lambda Science Artwork
27: Lambda Science Artwork
35: PHIL, Courtesy CDC

Cover: © Gary Gaugler/Visuals Unlimited

36: Lambda Science Artwork
44: Lambda Science Artwork
48: © CORBIS
57: © CORBIS
60: Lambda Science Artwork
66: Lambda Science Artwork
76: © Ted Streshinsky/CORBIS

About the Author

Dr. Donald Emmeluth spent most of his teaching career in upstate New York. An avid hiker and golfer, both endeavors provided him with ample opportunities to view the forests and grasslands of the countryside. In 1999, Dr. Emmeluth retired from the State University of New York system and moved to the warmer climate of Savannah, Georgia. He became a member of the Biology Department of Armstrong Atlantic State University (AASU) in Savannah. He continues to hike after golf balls on the various courses in and around Savannah and the Hilton Head, South Carolina, areas.

At AASU, Dr. Emmeluth teaches a course entitled Principles of Biology, Microbiology, Microorganisms, and Disease as well as a bioethics module that is part of the ethics course on campus. He developed and maintains the Biology Department website. Dr. Emmeluth has also published several journal articles and is the co-author of a high school biology textbook. His most recent article appeared in the February 2002 issue of *The American Biology Teacher*. The topic was bioinformatics. He has also authored another of the books in this series about Influenza. He has served as President of the National Association of Biology Teachers. During his career, Dr. Emmeluth has received a number of honors and awards including the Chancellor's Award for Excellence in Teaching and the Two-Year College Biology Teaching Award from NABT.

About the Editor

The late **I. Edward Alcamo** was a Distinguished Teaching Professor of Microbiology at the State University of New York at Farmingdale. Alcamo studied biology at Iona College in New York and earned his M.S. and Ph.D. degrees in microbiology at St. John's University, also in New York. He had taught at Farmingdale for over 30 years. In 2000, Alcamo won the Carski Award for Distinguished Teaching in Microbiology, the highest honor for microbiology teachers in the United States. He was a member of the American Society for Microbiology, the National Association of Biology Teachers, and the American Medical Writers Association. Alcamo authored numerous books on the subjects of microbiology, AIDS, and DNA technology as well as the award-winning textbook *Fundamentals of Microbiology*, now in its sixth edition.